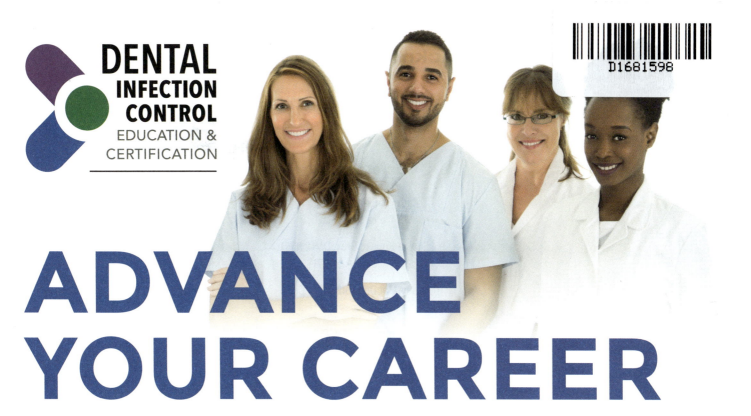

ADVANCE YOUR CAREER

Elevate your dental infection control expertise and demonstrate your commitment to patient safety through education and certification!

- OSAP-DALE Foundation Dental Infection Prevention and Control Certificate Program™ — A standardized dental infection control educational program

- Certified in Dental Infection Prevention and Control™ (CDIPC™)
  — A clinically-focused professional certification

- Dental Industry Specialist in Infection Prevention and Control™ (DISIPC™)
  — An industry (dental trade)-focused professional certification

Learn more at dentalinfectioncontrol.org.

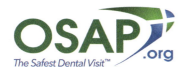 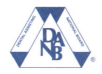 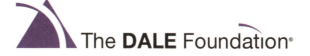

From Policy to Practice:

OSAP's Guide to the CDC Guidelines

Your tool for applying CDC dental infection prevention and control guidelines

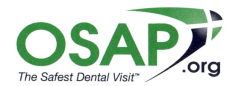

An education and training resource
prepared for dental healthcare personnel by OSAP —
the Organization for Safety, Asepsis and Prevention

From Policy to Practice: OSAP's Guide to the CDC Guidelines is an education and training tool produced by the Organization for Safety, Asepsis and Prevention (OSAP) and supported by Cooperative Agreement No. U58/CCU318566-02 from the U.S. Centers for Disease Control and Prevention. Its contents are solely the responsibility of OSAP and do not necessarily represent the official views of the Centers for Disease Control and Prevention.

Published by OSAP, Atlanta, GA.

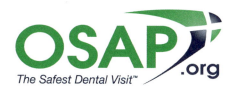

From Policy to Practice: OSAP's Guide to the CDC Guidelines

This workbook belongs to...

_____

In the practice setting belonging to...

_____

Training under the supervision of...

_____

Date training began:

_____

Date training was completed:

_____

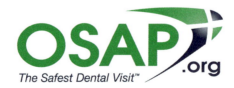

OSAP is the Organization for Safety, Asepsis and Prevention. Founded in 1984, the non-profit association is dentistry's premier resource for infection control and safety information. Through its publications, courses, website, and worldwide collaborations, OSAP and the tax-exempt OSAP Foundation support education, research, service, and policy development to promote safety and the control of infectious diseases in dental healthcare settings worldwide. For more information on OSAP activities, call (410)-571-0003 email office@osap.org, or visit osap.org.

From Policy to Practice: OSAP's Guide to the CDC Guidelines

Quick Start Guide to Using this Workbook

Who is OSAP?

The Organization for Safety, Asepsis and Prevention (OSAP) is a growing community of clinicians, consultants, educators, researchers, and industry representatives who advocate for safe and infection-free delivery of oral healthcare. OSAP focuses on strategies to improve compliance with safe practices and on building a strong network of recognized infection control experts.

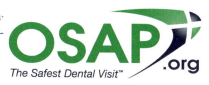

OSAP offers an extensive collection of resources, publications, FAQs, checklists and toolkits that help dental professionals deliver the safest dental visit possible for their patients. Plus, online and live courses help advance the level of knowledge and skill for every member of the dental team.

Who is CDC?

The Centers for Disease Control and Prevention (CDC) is the foremost public health agency in the United States. It reviews current scientific information and based on that information, creates recommendations to protect the health of the population at large. CDC also tracks disease trends across the country and may serve as primary investigator when disease outbreaks threaten public health. Using the information it gathers, the agency develops methods for preventing or limiting the occurrence of all diseases.

CDC recommendations set the standard for the infection control and safety practices used by dental professionals in the US. In 2003, CDC issued its Guidelines for Infection Control in Dental Health-Care Settings-2003. That document outlined specific recommendations for infection control and safety in dentistry and became the resource used by all dental practitioners.

In 2016, CDC revisited its Guidelines document and published *Summary of Infection Prevention Practices in Dental Settings: Basic Expectations for Safe Care*, a document that reinforced the existing guidelines, added some new recommendations, and provided checklists to help dental professionals implement and maintain the recommended practices.

Understanding and incorporating the CDC recommendations outlined in these two publications is essential to protecting dental staff and patients.

How is this workbook different from the CDC guidelines?

CDC's infection control guidelines outline only what dental workers (also called dental health care personnel (DHCP)) need to do, not how they can do it. Although this approach leaves plenty of room for professional judgment, it may not always provide all the information that DHCP need to comply with the recommendations.

From Policy to Practice: OSAP's Guide to the CDC Guidelines is designed to help you understand and implement the CDC guidelines. Although the CDC guidelines are comprehensive, they describe only what dental professionals should do, not how they should do it. For example, the CDC guidelines might specify that dental instruments be cleaned and then heat sterilized; the OSAP guide explains exactly how to clean and sterilize those instruments.

This OSAP guide will help you put the CDC guidelines into practice in your own setting. If you have questions while using this guide, talk to the infection control coordinator in your practice setting. There are also additional resources on the OSAP website: www.osap.org. Understanding and complying with all current CDC guidelines is essential to providing dental care that is safe for the patients and staff.

Getting the Most from this Workbook

From Policy to Practice: OSAP's Guide to the CDC Guidelines is written and organized with simplicity in mind. To best prepare yourself to learn the material in each chapter, follow this step-by-step guide to working through each chapter.

1 At the top right corner of each chapter's title page, you'll see a list of job categories. These identify — at minimum — the workers who will need to learn and comply with the information in that chapter.

Patient Care refers to Dentists, Hygienists, Assistants, and any others who directly provide care to patients.

Turnaround refers to staff responsible for instrument reprocessing as well as preparing the operatory before and after patient treatment.

Admin refers to Administrative staff such as the Receptionist, Other Office Staff, and those involved in recordkeeping.

Manager refers to the Employer, the Infection Control Coordinator, and depending on how job responsibilities are defined in your practice setting, possibly the Office Manager.

2 Down the right side of each chapter title page, there's a column titled "Terms You Should Know." This is very important. The words and phrases in this list will be used throughout the chapter to explain infection control concepts and procedures. Look up each term in the Glossary (beginning on page 166 of this workbook). When you are familiar with each term, you are ready to begin the chapter.

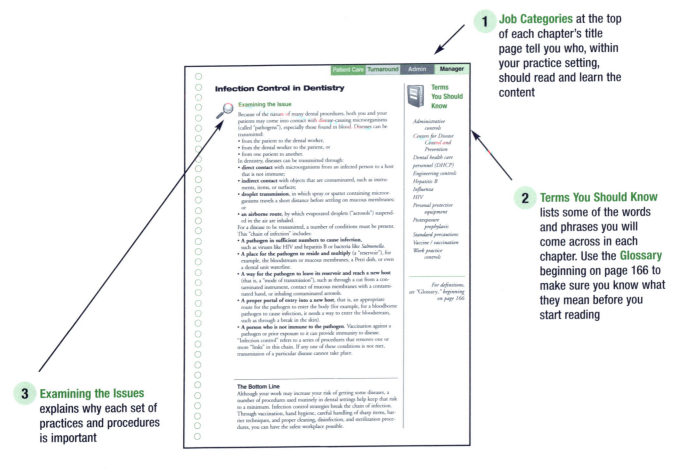

1 **Job Categories** at the top of each chapter's title page tell you who, within your practice setting, should read and learn the content

2 **Terms You Should Know** lists some of the words and phrases you will come across in each chapter. Use the **Glossary** beginning on page 166 to make sure you know what they mean before you start reading

3 **Examining the Issues** explains why each set of practices and procedures is important

3   To help you understand why you must apply each set of precautions in the dental setting, "Examining the Issues" provides a clear summary of the reasons behind recommended practices. The chapters also contain practical, step-by-step instructions, charts and checklists, pictures and captions, answers to common questions, and guidance in specific situations that require the use of clinical judgment. If you want to know about the science behind the recommendations, you can consult the actual CDC guidelines (available free of charge at *www.cdc.gov/oralhealth/infectioncontrol/guideline*.

4   With OSAP's "Exercises in Understanding," you work with your Infection Control Coordinator or Trainer to apply what you've learned in each chapter to your own practice setting).

5   A Self-Test at the end of each chapter helps make sure you're ready to move on to the next chapter. For any answers that you miss, reread the section and take any questions to your Infection Control Coordinator.

6   If you need more information, "Recommended Readings and Resources" can point you in the right direction.

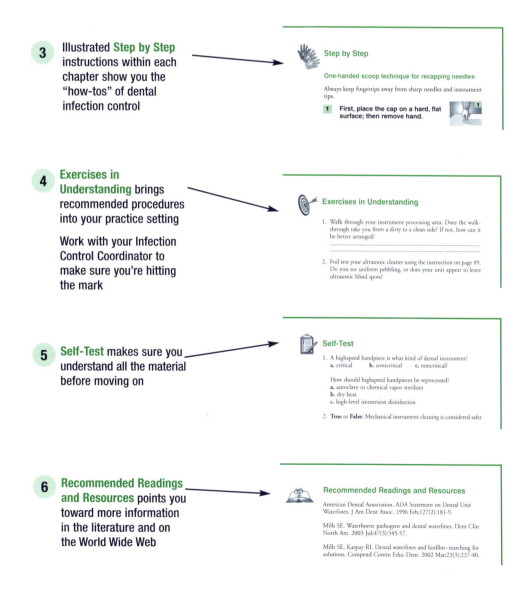

3 Illustrated **Step by Step** instructions within each chapter show you the "how-tos" of dental infection control

Step by Step

One-handed scoop technique for recapping needles

Always keep fingertips away from sharp needles and instrument tips.

1 First, place the cap on a hard, flat surface; then remove hand.

4 **Exercises in Understanding** brings recommended procedures into your practice setting

Work with your Infection Control Coordinator to make sure you're hitting the mark

Exercises in Understanding

1. Walk through your instrument processing area. Does the walk-through take you from a dirty to a clean side? If not, how can it be better arranged?

2. Foil test your ultrasonic cleaner using the instruction on page 49. Do you see uniform pebbling, or does your unit appear to leave ultrasonic blind spots?

5 **Self-Test** makes sure you understand all the material before moving on

Self-Test

1. A highspeed handpiece is what kind of dental instrument?
   a. critical   **b.** semicritical   **c.** noncritical?

   How should highspeed handpieces be reprocessed?
   a. autoclave or chemical vapor sterilizer
   b. dry heat
   c. high-level immersion disinfection

2. **True** or **False**: Mechanical instrument cleaning is considered safer

6 **Recommended Readings and Resources** points you toward more information in the literature and on the World Wide Web

Recommended Readings and Resources

American Dental Association. ADA Statement on Dental Unit Waterlines. J Am Dent Assoc. 1996 Feb;127(2):181-9.

Mills SE. Waterborne pathogens and dental waterlines. Dent Clin North Am. 2003 Jul;47(3):545-57.

Mills SE, Karpay RI. Dental waterlines and biofilm--searching for solutions. Compend Contin Educ Dent. 2002 Mar;23(3):237-40,

Chapter 1

An Introduction to Dental Infection Control

Examining the Issues

Healthcare-Associated Infections

While patients are receiving healthcare, they can be infected by germs unrelated to their treatment. Known as healthcare-associated infections, or HAIs, these infections occur in hospitals, medical and dental offices, urgent care centers, dialysis centers, nursing homes and any other setting where healthcare is delivered. HAIs can spread in many ways. For example, some patients are infected from contaminated or improperly used equipment while others are infected from the unclean hands of a healthcare worker.

When HAIs occur, the cause is often traced to a failure to follow recommended prevention practices. In 2015, after several alarming media reports of people being notified that they were treated with contaminated medical devices, CDC issued an official health advisory* to address the critical public health need for proper maintenance, cleaning, disinfection or sterilization of medical devices. This CDC health advisory also highlighted the importance of following guidelines to prevent infections in healthcare settings, including the continued education and training of healthcare workers in infection prevention and control.

Healthcare Workers

Healthcare workers, also called healthcare personnel (HCP), include all people working (paid or unpaid) in health-care settings who may have exposure to patients or infectious materials. Some examples of healthcare workers include dental workers as well as physicians, nurses, assistants, therapists, technicians, emergency personnel, pharmacists, and laboratory personnel. It may surprise you that healthcare workers also include students and trainees, volunteers, contractors, and people not directly involved in patient care but might be exposed to infectious agents. When healthcare workers are infected while doing their jobs, it is often referred to as an occupational illness.

Dental Workers are Healthcare Workers

Also called dental health care personnel (DHCP), dental workers include all paid or unpaid people working in dental care settings who might be exposed to infectious materials such as body substances, contaminated medical supplies and equipment, contaminated environmental surfaces, or contaminated water or air. This includes dentists, dental hygienists, dental assistants, students and trainees, dental laboratory technicians, contractors, and volunteers. DHCP also include people who do not participate in direct patient care, but are potentially exposed to infectious agents, such as administrative, clerical, housekeeping, maintenance personnel, and visiting sales representatives.

*Centers for Disease Control and Prevention Health Advisory: Immediate Need for Healthcare Facilities to Review Procedures for Cleaning, Disinfecting and Sterilizing Reusable Medical Devices. HAN382 Sept 11, 2015. emergency.cdc.gov/han/han00382.asp ; Updated Oct 2, 2015. HAN383; Updated Oct 2, 2015. HAN383 emergency.cdc.gov/han/han00383.asp

The Bottom Line

As a dental worker, you are an important member of the healthcare team. By learning and following safe practices and infection control techniques, both you and your patients can have the safest dental visit possible.

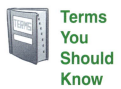

Terms You Should Know

Aerosols

Bloodborne pathogen

Chain of infection

Contaminated / Contamination

Direct contact

Host

Healthcare-associated infection

Immunity

Indirect contact

Microorganism

Mode of transmission

Occupational exposure

Pathogen

Personal protective equipment

Spatter

Standard precautions

Universal precautions

For definitions, see "Glossary," beginning on page 166

Diseases and Modes of Transmission in the Dental Setting

A number of diseases can be transmitted via routine dental care. Fortunately, infection control and safety procedures such as hand-washing, personal protective equipment, injury prevention techniques, and proper care of items and surfaces greatly reduce the risk to patients and DHCP.

Bloodborne
Hepatitis B
Hepatitis C
Human immunodeficiency virus (HIV)

Contact
Chickenpox
Hepatitis A
Herpes

Droplet
Mumps
Rubella
Influenza

Airborne
Chickenpox
Measles
Tuberculosis

Disease Transmission

Because of the nature of many dental procedures, both you and your patients may come into contact with disease-causing microorganisms (called "pathogens"), especially those found in blood. Diseases can be transmitted through:

○ **direct contact** with microorganisms from an infected person to a host that is not immune;
○ **indirect contact** with objects that are contaminated, such as instruments, items, or surfaces;
○ **droplet transmission**, in which spray or spatter containing microorganisms travels a short distance before settling on mucous membranes; or
○ **an airborne route**, by which evaporated droplets ("aerosols") suspended in the air are inhaled.

For a disease to be transmitted, a number of conditions must be present. This "chain of infection" includes:
○ **A pathogen in sufficient numbers to cause infection**, such as viruses like HIV and hepatitis B or bacteria like *Salmonella*.
○ **A place for the pathogen to reside and multiply** (a "reservoir"), for example, the bloodstream or mucous membranes, a Petri dish, or even a dental unit waterline.
○ **A way for the pathogen to leave its reservoir and reach a new host** (that is, a "mode of transmission"), such as through a cut from a contaminated instrument, contact of mucous membranes with a contaminated hand, or inhaling contaminated aerosols.
○ **A proper portal of entry into a new host**, that is, an appropriate route for the pathogen to enter the body (for example, for a bloodborne pathogen to cause infection, it needs a way to enter the bloodstream, such as through a break in the skin).
○ **A person who is not immune to the pathogen**. Vaccination against a pathogen or prior exposure to it can provide immunity to disease.

Infection control also called **infection prevention** refers to a series of procedures that removes one or more "links" in this chain. If any one of these conditions is not met, transmission of a particular disease cannot take place.

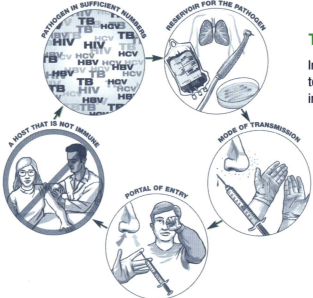

The 'Chain of Infection'

Infection control attempts to break one or more "links" in the chain of infection.

Principles of Infection Control

Applying the four basic principles of infection control will guide you in keeping yourself and your patients safe.

1. Take action to stay healthy.
Your first obligation to yourself and your patients is to stay healthy. Remember that a susceptible host must be present for infection to occur; if you are not susceptible, you cannot acquire (and therefore can't transmit) a disease. Get vaccinated against hepatitis B and other vaccine preventable diseases.

2. Avoid contact with blood and body fluids.
A number of potentially serious diseases are spread through blood; other diseases are spread through contact with other body fluids. There is no way to know for certain which patients are infected. As such, avoid direct contact with blood, body fluids, non-intact skin, and mucous membranes. Always use standard precautions — handwashing; gloves, eyewear and face protection; controls to prevent injuries — and treat every patient as if infectious.

3. Limit the spread of blood and body fluid contamination.
Blood and other patient materials can be spread in many ways: through spatter created during dental procedures, by touching supplies, equipment, and furniture with contaminated hands, or by laying a contaminated instrument on a clean surface. Any item or area that you contaminate becomes a potential source of exposure. By taking care not to spread contamination, you help yourself and others avoid contact with blood and other potentially infectious body fluids.

4. Make objects safe for use.
Even doing your best to control the spread of blood or other body fluids, some instruments, items, equipment, and surfaces become contaminated during patient treatment. Always clean, package, then sterilize instruments before they are used again. Likewise, before seating the next patient, clean then disinfect or cover with a surface barrier any unprotected surfaces that became contaminated.

Principles of Infection Control...In Action

Take action to stay healthy	Limit the spread of contamination
• Get immunized • Report occupational injuries and exposures immediately • Follow the advice of the medical care provider evaluating your occupational exposure	• Set up the operatory before starting treatment; unit-dose supplies • Cover surfaces that will be contaminated • Minimize splashes and spatter • Properly dispose of all waste
Avoid contacting blood / body fluids	**Make objects safe for use**
• Wear gloves, protective clothing, and face and eye protection • Handle sharps with care • Use safety devices as appropriate • Use mechanical devices to clean instruments whenever possible	• Know the different decontamination processes • Read chemical germicide labels • Monitor processes to make sure they're working as they should

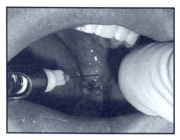

The nature of many dental procedures puts workers in close contact with patients' blood and oral fluids.

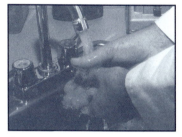

Handwashing is an important part of infection control. Washing your hands can help keep you healthy.

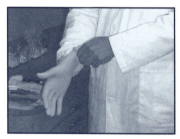

Wear personal protective equipment to prevent contact with body fluids.

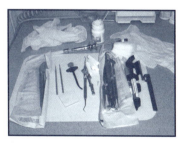

Set out supplies before treatment so you won't need to touch containers or cabinets with contaminated hands.

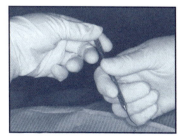

Pass sharp instruments with the tips away from all persons to minimize the risk of injury.

A Dental Health Care Personnel's Greatest Risk

Although you may be aware that HIV, the virus that causes acquired immunodeficiency syndrome (AIDS), is a bloodborne disease risk, you may not know that it is not the greatest risk to a DHCP. In fact, the most transmissible bloodborne agent is not HIV, but HBV — the hepatitis B virus.

Infection with hepatitis B virus is a major health problem that can cause lifelong infection, scarring of the liver, liver cancer, liver failure, and death.

HBV is usually transmitted during contact with blood. Healthcare workers, including DHCP, may become infected when exposed to an infected patient's blood, typically through a stick or cut with a sharp instrument, or through spatter contacting their eyes, nose, or mouth. Getting patient blood on cuts and cracks in skin also may cause infection.

As a DHCP, you have an increased risk of contact with blood and body fluids and are more likely to become infected with HBV than most people. Fortunately, a vaccine is available. If you have not been immunized against hepatitis B virus, talk to your Infection Control Coordinator about getting vaccinated today. For more info, see Ch. 2, Elements of a Dental Personnel Health Program

Universal Precautions

Universal precautions are infection control and safety procedures to protect against bloodborne disease transmission. Because patients with bloodborne infections may not appear sick or may not be aware that they are infected, universal precautions assume that all blood, and any body fluid that might be contaminated with blood (such as saliva), is infectious.

Standard Precautions

Standard precautions expand the concept of universal precautions beyond exposure to blood and represent a standard of care designed to protect HCP and patients from pathogens that can be spread by:

- blood
- all body fluids, secretions, and excretions (except sweat)
- non-intact skin
- mucous membranes

Standard precautions are applied to all patient care, in any healthcare setting, regardless of whether a patient has a suspected or confirmed infection. Standard precautions include—

- Hand hygiene
- Use of personal protective equipment
- Cleaning and disinfecting environmental surfaces
- Safe injection practices and sharps safety
- Sterilization of instruments and devices
- Respiratory hygiene/cough etiquette

Respiratory hygiene/cough etiquette and safe injection practices were added to standard precautions in 2007 and are critical elements of any infection control program. For a list of all CDC dental infection control recommendations, including new items relevant to dentistry since 2003, see Appendix A of this workbook.

Transmission-Based Precautions

For patients with highly infectious diseases that are easily spread through skin contact, or through airborne or droplet routes, the risk of spreading infection may require standard precautions to be supplemented with another tier of protection called transmission-based precautions. Although dental offices are not usually equipped for the level of isolation required for using transmission-based precautions, sick patients requiring this level of precaution usually do not come in for routine dental care. However, your infection control program should include a plan to detect and manage potentially infectious patients as soon as they enter your facility. Consider rescheduling non-urgent dental care until such patients are no longer infectious. Alternatively, when urgent dental care is necessary, refer infectious patients that require transmission-based precautions to a facility that can provide treatment using appropriate isolation practices.

Respiratory Hygiene / Cough Etiquette

When patients arrive sick, or if people who arrive with them are sick, they can spread infection to others in the waiting area, restrooms, front desk or other parts of your dental facility. Respiratory Hygiene/Cough Etiquette, an important part of standard precautions, applies to any patient or staff member who shows signs of respiratory illness such as a cough, congestion or runny nose. Your dental practice should have a system in place to detect and manage potentially infectious persons soon after they arrive at your facility.

CDC recommends the following actions for respiratory hygiene/cough etiquette:

- Implementing measures to contain respiratory secretions in patients and accompanying individuals who have signs and symptoms of a respiratory infection, beginning at point of entry to the facility and continuing through the visit
- Posting signs with instructions for:
  - Covering mouth/nose when coughing or sneezing.
  - Using and discarding tissues.
  - Cleaning hands after coming in contact with respiratory secretions.

- Providing tissues and no-touch trash bins.
- Providing resources for hand hygiene in or near waiting areas.
- Offering masks to people with a runny nose, cough or other signs of respiratory illness when they enter your facility.
- Providing space and encouraging people with symptoms of respiratory infections to sit away from others.
- Educating staff on the importance of ways to prevent the spread of respiratory germs from patients with signs and symptoms of a respiratory infection.

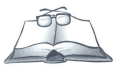

Recommended Readings and Resources

Molinari JA, Harte, JA eds. *Practical Infection Control in Dentistry,* 3rd edition. Philadelphia: Lippincott, Williams & Wilkins, 2010.

Miller CH,. *Infection Control and Management of Hazardous Materials for the Dental Team,* 6th edition. St. Louis: Elsevier, 2018

Harte JA. Standard and Transmission Based Precautions: *An update for Dentistry. JADA 141(5):572-581; 2010*

OSAP. If Saliva Were Red: A Visual Lesson on Infection Control. *www.osap.org*

Centers for Disease Control and Prevention. *Summary of Infection Prevention Practices in Dental Settings: Basic Expectations for Safe Care. 2016. www.cdc.gov/oralhealth/infection-control/pdf/safe-care2.pdf*

Centers for Disease Control and Prevention. *2007 Guideline for Isolation Precautions: Preventing Transmission of Infectious Agents in Healthcare Settings. www.cdc.gov/infectioncontrol/guide lines/isolation/index.html*

Centers for Disease Control and Prevention. *Management of Multidrug-Resistant Organisms in Healthcare Settings, 2006. www.cdc.gov/infectioncontrol/guide lines/mdro/index.html*

Universal Precautions and Standard Precautions

	Procedures include...	To protect against exposure to...
Universal Precautions	• Hand hygiene • Personal protective equipment (gloves, eyewear, and face protection) • Controls to prevent injuries • Proper management of patient care items and environmental surfaces	Blood, some other body fluids
Standard Precautions	• Hand hygiene • Personal protective equipment (gloves, eyewear, and face protection) • Respiratory hygiene/cough etiquette • Safe injection practices and sharps safety • Sterilization of instruments and devices • Cleaning and disinfecting environmental surfaces	Blood, body secretions, excretions, nonintact skin, mucous membranes

The Infection Control Plan

Every dental office should have a written infection control plan and have enough resources available to develop and maintain an infection control program. This includes providing training and supplies to ensure the safety of patients and staff. At least one person among your staff should be trained to serve as the Infection Control Coordinator and maintain the overall coordination, management and assessment of the infection control program.

The Infection Control Plan Should:
- Be developed, written and maintained to align with the type of dental services provided by your facility.
- Include written policies and procedures developed from infection control guide-lines, regulations or standards that go beyond Occupational Safety and Health Administration (OSHA) bloodborne pathogens training.
- Be reviewed annually and revised from new recommendations, new safety products, and state and/or federal requirements or regulations.
- Be managed by someone who is trained in infection control and serves as the Infection Control Coordinator.
- Ensure that the correct supplies are available to follow Standard Precautions.
- Describe ways to detect and manage, as soon as possible, potentially infectious persons that come into your facility.

Common Questions and Answers

How are microorganisms spread in the dental operatory?

Direct transmission can occur via person-to-person contact, via droplets that are produced through sneezing or coughing, or by spatter during dental procedures. Microorganisms also can be spread indirectly or by airborne routes.

What is indirect transmission?

In indirect transmission, microorganisms are first transferred to an object, such as an instrument or surface, and then transferred to another person.

What is airborne transmission?

With airborne transmission, microorganisms from an infected person become suspended in air, where they can be inhaled by others when they breathe. Some microorganisms, such as those that cause chickenpox, measles, or tuberculosis, can be spread by airborne transmission. Bloodborne microorganisms, including those that cause AIDS and hepatitis B, are not transmitted in this way.

What is bloodborne transmission?

Bloodborne transmission is the transfer of bloodborne pathogens from an infected host to a susceptible person. This can occur through cuts, puncture wounds, or cracks in the skin, or by splashes to the mucous membranes that allow an infected person's blood to enter the new person's bloodstream.

Exercises in Understanding

1. On a separate sheet of paper, write down the four principles of infection control and what they mean to you. Compare your answers with those described earlier in this chapter.
2. Cite examples of some of the ways you expect to apply each principle in your practice setting. Share your responses with your Infection Control Manager.

Self-Test

Before moving on, test yourself with some questions on the material. (answers appear below)

1. What events are necessary for infection to occur?

   _____

   _____

   _____

2. While working in a dental office, how can you become infected with a bloodborne pathogen?

   _____

   _____

3. What disease poses the greatest risk of infection to dental health care personnel?

   _____

(1) All of the following: pathogen in sufficient numbers; reservoir in which the pathogen can survive and multiply; mode of transmission; portal of entry in a new, susceptible host. (2) Through cuts, puncture wounds, or cracks in the skin, or by splashes to the mucous membranes that allow an infected person's blood to enter your bloodstream. (3) Hepatitis B.

Chapter 2

Elements of a Dental Personnel Health Program

Examining the Issues

To help protect your health and safety while on the job and in turn, the health and safety of your patients, your work setting should have an occupational health program. Your Infection Control Coordinator can familiarize you with all the actions taken to ensure your health and safety.

Remember: Protecting your occupational health also protects your overall health, so do what you can to comply with your practice setting's recommendations for keeping safe at work.

Your practice setting should have:

○ A written personnel health service program for DHCP that addresses:
  ❏ education and training;
  ❏ immunization programs;
  ❏ exposure prevention and postexposure management;
  ❏ medical conditions, work-related illness, and work restrictions;
  ❏ latex hypersensitivity and other work-associated skin reactions; and
  ❏ maintenance of records, data management, and confidentiality.

○ A referral arrangement with qualified medical professionals to ensure that any necessary job-related medical evaluation and treatment can be delivered quickly and appropriately (see Ch. 3, Preventing Transmission of Bloodborne Pathogens).

○ An education and training schedule that provides training on infection control procedures specific to your duties and responsibilities. You should receive this training before you begin performing any duties that put you at risk of exposure to body fluids as well as periodically thereafter.

○ A written immunization program that outlines:
  ❏ all required and recommended vaccinations/immunizations for staff by job title/description, and
  ❏ referral to a healthcare professional to receive appropriate vaccinations.

○ Written work restriction and exclusion policies in your workplace (including who may implement restrictions and exclusions).

○ A confidential, up-to-date medical record for all workers, maintained and stored either onsite or with your practice's healthcare professional/facility. Records should only include documentation of immunization and of any tests received as a result of an occupational exposure.

You should be trained in:

○ Administrative, engineering, and work practice controls that reduce your risk of contracting an illness or sustaining an injury while doing your job.

○ Policies and procedures for prompt reporting of injuries and obtaining appropriate medical evaluation and followup care (see Ch. 3).

○ The importance of reporting any medical conditions or medical treatments that may make you more susceptible to injury or infection, or that may create a significant risk of transmission to other staff members and patients.

The Bottom Line

Both you and your employer must work together to ensure your safety and the safety of all the patients you treat. Continual education and training, combined with your willingness to use proper infection control procedures in practice, can increase your safety, the safety of your patients, and even your community.

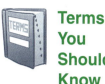

Terms You Should Know

Administrative controls

Confidentiality

Engineering controls

Exposure prevention

Exposure management

Immunization

Infection Control Coordinator

Latex hypersensitivity

Medical records

Occupational injury

Occupational illness

Qualified healthcare professional

Vaccination / vaccine

Work practice controls

Work restrictions/ exclusions

For definitions, see "Glossary," beginning on page 166

Recommended Immunizations for DHCP

The U.S. Public Health Service recommends that DHCP be vaccinated against the following illnesses:

- Hepatitis B
- Influenza
- Measles
- Mumps
- Rubella
- Tetanus, with a booster every 10 years
- Varicella-zoster (chickenpox)

For more info, see Appendix C, p.154

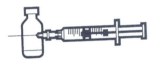

Tetanus Booster

Td is the abbreviation for the tetanus-diptheria vaccine given to adults as a booster every 10 years, or sometimes after an exposure to tetanus. Tdap is another tetanus vaccine, but also protects against diphtheria and pertussis.

You can have Tdap no matter when you last got a Td booster shot. All healthcare workers who have not, or are not sure if they've had a dose of Tdap should get a dose of Tdap as soon as possible. Female healthcare workers should get Tdap during each pregnancy.

Vaccines and Dental Health Care Personnel: The Facts

○ **Healthcare workers are at risk of acquiring diseases through their work.** In addition to bloodborne diseases such as hepatitis B and hepatitis C, unvaccinated healthcare workers also are at risk of catching or transmitting diseases like influenza ("the flu"), measles, mumps, rubella, and chickenpox (varicella).

○ **Getting vaccinated before you are placed at risk** is the most efficient and effective way to protect your health.

○ **All healthcare workers should receive the vaccines recommended by the U.S. Public Health Service** Advisory Committee on Immunization Practices (ACIP). See Appendix C, p.154

○ **Workers who do not directly provide patient care but come into contact with patients or patient materials also should be vaccinated** (for example, administrators and lab personnel).

Common Questions & Answers

If I get vaccinated, I will never get infected, right?

No vaccine is 100% effective, but most come close. CDC reports that the measles vaccine is about 97% effective and influenza vaccination can reduce the risk of flu illness by about 40-60% overall.

Today's vaccines are very safe. Most side effects are minor and temporary, such as a sore arm or a mild fever. Taking an over-the-counter pain reliever/fever reducer before and after vaccination can help with these symptoms.

Before receiving any vaccine, however, be sure to give the healthcare provider a full medical history, including any allergies.

How can I obtain the recommended vaccines?

Your employer should have arranged for a healthcare professional or facility to manage the occupational medical needs of the workers in your practice setting. Speak with your Infection Control Coordinator for details.

My office does not have a medical provider/facility to handle our occupational health needs. How can we find one?

Good choices for your practice's medical facility include an infectious disease specialist or an occupational medical center (these facilities often are associated with universities or teaching hospitals). Both can handle recommended vaccinations and should be well-versed and current in managing occupational injuries and other exposures.

Be sure to get information on where to go for after-hours exposure management. As you will read in Ch. 3, timing of injury evaluation and management is critical. An exposure is a medical emergency. Exposures that happen on Saturday morning can't wait until Monday; they need to be managed *now*.

Include the name and contact information of the medical provider in your training materials and exposure control plan, and be sure to have maps and directions handy to save time in getting to the treatment facility.

Exercises in Understanding

1. Indicate with a checkmark in the appropriate column what your status is for each disease listed below.

Disease	1. Immunized and up to date	2. Have had the disease	3. Not immunized or not up to date	4. Have not had the disease	5. Don't know
Hepatitis B (3 dose series)					
Influenza (annually)					
Measles					
Mumps					
Rubella					
Tetanus (every 10 years)					
Varicella zoster (chickenpox)					

2. If you did not check either column 1 or 2 for any disease above, discuss the need for vaccination updates with your physician.

3. Where do you and your coworkers go for occupational health needs such as vaccinations and injury management?

   Name of doctor/facility: _____

   Address/phone number: _____

4. What is the training schedule in your practice setting? _____
   When are you due for your next periodic review? _____

Self-Test

Before moving on, test yourself with some questions on the material.
(answers appear below)

1. A tetanus booster is recommended every _____ year(s).
   a. 1   b. 3   c. 5   d. 10

2. The most efficient and effective way to protect your health is:
   a. vaccination   c. gloves, masks, and eyewear
   b. using safety devices   d. eating healthy

3. Name four vaccine-preventable diseases you should be immunized against.

   _____   _____

   _____   _____

4. Training must be provided:
   a. when you first start your job   c. on your own time
   b. periodically thereafter   d. both a and b

(1) d; (2) a; (3) any of the following you've received: Hepatitis B, influenza, measles, mumps, rubella, tetanus, varicella-zoster (chickenpox); (4) d

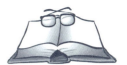

Recommended Readings and Resources

Centers for Disease Control and Prevention. Recommended vaccines for healthcare workers. www.cdc.gov/vaccines/adults/rec-vac/hcw.html

Centers for Disease Control and Prevention. Influenza Vaccination of Health-Care Personnel. Recommendations of the Healthcare Infection Control Practices Advisory Committee (HICPAC) and the Advisory Committee on Immunization Practices (ACIP). Available at *www.cdc.gov/MMWR/preview/mmwrhtml/rr5502a1.htm?c_cid=journal_search_promotion_2018*

Centers for Disease Control and Prevention. Influenza Vaccination Information for Health Care Workers, available at:www.cdc.gov/flu/healthcareworkers.htm

Eklund KJ, Bednarsh H, Haaland CO. OSHA and CDC Guidelines. OSAP Interact Training System. *www.osap.org*

Occupational Safety & Health Administration (OSHA). Bloodborne Pathogens and Needlestick Prevention Standards, available at: *www.osha.gov/SLTC/bloodbornepathogens/index.html*

OSAP. Plotting a Course to Infection Prevention Through Immunization. *Infection Control in Practice. October 2013;12(5);1-4.*

Notes

Chapter 3

Preventing Transmission of Bloodborne Pathogens

 ## Examining the Issues

Bloodborne pathogens are disease agents that exist in blood and certain body fluids of infected individuals. Examples include hepatitis B virus (HBV), hepatitis C virus (HCV), and the human immunodeficiency virus (HIV).

Under certain circumstances, these disease agents can be transmitted from patient to DHCP, from DHCP to patient, and from patient to patient through exposure to infected blood or other body fluids. Exposures occur through percutaneous injury (e.g., a needlestick or cut with a sharp object) as well as through contact between potentially infectious blood, tissues, or other body fluids and mucous membranes of the eyes, nose, mouth, or nonintact skin (e.g., exposed skin that is chapped or broken).

The most effective ways to prevent transmission of bloodborne pathogens include vaccination against HBV infection, standard precautions, and strategies to prevent injuries with sharp instruments.

Strategies to prevent injuries include:
○ **Engineering controls**. Some devices used in the dental setting are specifically designed to prevent or reduce exposure to blood and body fluids. These engineering controls rely on the device's technology, rather than the user's technique, to reduce the likelihood of an injury that could transmit a disease. Engineering controls include safer versions of sharp devices, mechanical instrument washers, needle recappers, and sharps containers.
○ **Work practice controls**. Some work practices are safer than others. For example, using the one-handed scoop technique to recap needles (described on p. 15) is a work practice control that is safer than recapping a contaminated needle using two hands.
○ **Personal protective equipment**. By creating a physical barrier between you and the patient, personal protective equipment such as gloves, face protection, and protective apparel helps prevent exposures to blood and body fluids.

 ## The Bottom Line

Transmission of bloodborne pathogens in dental settings occurs infrequently but can have serious consequences. Hepatitis B vaccination and strategies to prevent exposures to blood are the key to protecting yourself, your coworkers, and the patients you treat.

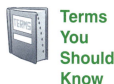 ## Terms You Should Know

Bloodborne pathogens
Carrier
Cross-contamination
Culture of Safety
Engineering controls
Hepatitis B virus
Hepatitis C virus
HIV / AIDS
Immunity
Other potentially infectious materials (OPIM)
Percutaneous injury
Personal protective equipment
Portal of entry
Seroconversion
Source patient
Standard precautions
Virus
Work practice controls

For definitions, see "Glossary," beginning on page 166

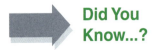

Did You Know...?

○ **Persons with hepatitis C can be infected for more than 20 years before they start feeling the symptoms of their infection**.

○ **Some persons who carry the hepatitis B virus may show no signs of disease themselves but may be highly infectious to others** who come into contact with their blood and body fluids. These persons are called "carriers."

○ **Many individuals who are HIV-positive may not be aware that they are infected.**

○ **Standard precautions demands that all patients be treated as if they are carrying an infectious disease.** That is, the same means of protecting against exposures and cross-contamination must be used for each and every patient.

○ **Vaccination against hepatitis B virus offers the best protection against the bloodborne disease**. Get vaccinated before you're placed at risk.

Bloodborne Disease Facts

Hepatitis B ...

○ **... is very infectious.** HBV can survive on surfaces for at least 7 - 10 days and can be transmitted even when blood is not visible.

○ **... is a serious, well-recognized occupational risk for DHCP**, but DHCP getting vaccinated and using standard precautions has helped to dramatically decrease the rate of work-acquired infections.

○ **... is best combatted through vaccination**. More than 90% of U.S. dentists have been vaccinated against hepatitis B. For unvaccinated DHCP who have been exposed to blood or other infectious body fluids, postexposure management calls for use of the vaccine and, when indicated, an injection (shot) of immune globulin to reduce the risk of getting the disease.

Hepatitis C ...

○ **... now kills more Americans than any other infectious disease.** However, highly effective treatments are now available that may cure HCV infections.

○ **... is not easily transmitted through occupational exposures**, but some risk may exist. Based on limited studies, CDC reports that the estimated risk for infection after a needlestick or cut exposure to HCV-infected blood is approximately 1.8%.

○ **... has no vaccine at this time.**

Human Immunodeficiency Virus (HIV)...

○ **... is the virus that causes AIDS** (Acquired Immune Deficiency Syndrome).

○ **... transmission risk in dental settings is extremely low**. As of December 2001, no DHCP is known to have become HIV-positive following a documented occupational exposure to an infected patient's blood or body fluids. Although six patients in Florida are believed to have become infected with HIV through dental care, those cases happened about 30 years ago and all were associated with care from the same HIV-positive dentist. How transmission occurred was never determined, even after extensive investigation by public health agencies. Of the millions of dental procedures performed each year, those six cases are the only ones associated with dental care in the history of HIV/AIDS.

○ **... infection may be prevented with postexposure prophylaxis, but medication must be started very quickly after exposure.** Administered within 1 to 2 hours of exposure, some drugs can significantly reduce the risk of disease transmission.

○ **... has no vaccine at this time.**

Hepatitis B virus is the DHCP's greatest occupational risk. Fortunately, a vaccine is available.

Getting Immunized Against Hepatitis B

Steps to Immunity

1. Get Vaccination series (3 doses)

↓

2. Get Tested for Antibodies

If antibodies are present, you're protected

If antibodies are not detected, undergo a second 3-dose series of injections

↓

Get tested for antibodies
1-2 months after the third dose

↓

If antibodies are not detected...

↓

Undergo further blood testing

You may have protection from a previous hepatitis B infection, you may be a carrier, or you may still be susceptible to infection

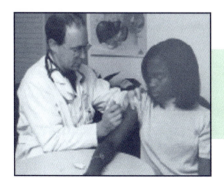

Immunization is the best protection against disease.

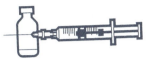

In dentistry, workers can suffer injuries and exposures to blood and blood-contaminated saliva. Protective barriers cannot eliminate all potential exposures, so vaccination remains the best protection against infection.

What vaccines protect against bloodborne pathogens in dentistry?

The hepatitis B vaccine is available and recommended for all workers involved in direct patient care. It is given in 3 injections, preferably in the upper arm. There are currently no vaccines for hepatitis C virus or HIV.

Is the hepatitis B vaccine safe?

The vaccines available today use only non-infectious virus particles, so for the vast majority of people, they are very safe and effective. Because of some other vaccine components, people who are allergic to yeast should not receive the vaccine. Your medical professional can give you more info.

How long does HBV immunity last?

About 95% of healthy, properly vaccinated young adults develop protective antibodies to the virus. Protection lasts at least 15 years. Boosters are not recommended at this time.

BIOHAZARD

Identifying Biohazards

A biohazard refers to a biological agent or a condition that poses a threat to humans. In dentistry, the agent is typically an infectious microorganism, and the condition would be contamination with such microorganisms.

The universal biohazard symbol (⚕) is your warning of an infectious hazard. Usually appearing on an orange or red background, this symbol indicates a potential for exposure and signals the need for appropriate precautions.

You will see this symbol on:

❑ containers of regulated waste,
❑ refrigerators or freezers containing blood or other potentially infectious materials that may contain blood-borne pathogens,
❑ contaminated laundry containers,
❑ sharps containers,
❑ anywhere else an infectious hazard exists.

The color red also may be used to denote a biohazard. Hence, the term "red bagging" contaminated laundry and regulated waste.

Precautions to Avoid Exposures to Blood

Some common-sense advice for reducing your risk of exposure to blood and body fluids:

Stay Aware

○ Consider items that are contaminated with patient blood and saliva as potentially infectious. Handle sharp items with care to prevent injuries. Sharps items in dentistry include needles, scalpel blades, wires, and many hand instruments.
○ Remember: Every patient you treat could be carrying an infectious disease. Always use standard precautions to protect yourself and your patients.
○ Know the details of your practice's sharps injury prevention program and whom to contact in case of accidental exposures.

Use engineering controls, for example:

○ Screen and evaluate sharps safety devices for use in your practice as they become available. Use appropriate, effective devices with safety features, such as safety syringes, retractable scalpels, and needleless IV ports. When used correctly, these devices may help reduce injuries (for example, some safety syringes replace the need to recap needles between injections on the same patient).
○ Use devices that minimize handling of contaminated items and in turn, the risk of injury. Needle recappers, ultrasonic cleaners, and instrument cassettes are common examples in the dental office.
○ Use leakproof, puncture-resistant sharps containers to discard disposable syringes and needles, scalpel blades, and other sharp items. Make sure your sharps containers are color-coded red or labeled with the biohazard symbol. They also should have a visible "fill to" line, and you should be able to see how full the container is without having to place a sharp item inside. Sharps containers should have a seal that securely closes to prevent spills during transport. Place sharps containers in each operatory near the point of use and wherever else contaminated sharps are handled.

Use safer work practices, for example:

○ Never use two hands to recap a needle. The one-handed "scoop" technique or a recapping device reduces the potential for injuries.
○ Place contaminated sharps in sharps containers as soon as possible after use. Keep sharps containers near the point of use (for example, in each operatory), and replace them before they are overfilled.
○ Pass instruments with sharp ends pointing away from all persons, and announce instrument passes so the receiving DHCP knows a sharp object is coming into his or her workspace.
○ Use instruments instead of fingers to retract tissues during suturing and anesthetic injections.

Wear personal protective equipment whenever exposure to patient body fluids is expected.

○ Wear gloves, face protection, eye protection, and protective clothing as described in Ch. 5, Personal Protective Equipment.

Learn and routinely apply exposure-prevention techniques as outlined in your practice.

○ Be familiar with your facility's written, comprehensive program for minimizing and managing worker exposure to blood and other potentially infectious body fluids.

Sharps Safety and Your Injury Prevention Program

Your practice setting's injury prevention program should include a process to identify, screen, and evaluate safer dental devices. Routinely use devices that appear safer than the traditional sharps. The Centers for Disease Control and Prevention (CDC) has developed sample forms for screening and evaluating safer sharps devices for dentistry. See Appendix E, p.159 of this workbook.

A successful sharps safety program as a part of your practice's culture of safety will:

❍ ensure that the dental team actively works to maintain a safe workplace;

❍ encourage prompt reporting and postexposure injury management;

❍ identify and intervene to eliminate unsafe work practices and devices;

❍ coordinate annually, safety device selection, screening and evaluation;

❍ organize staff education and training;

❍ keep the necessary records; and

❍ monitor safety performance and gather staff feedback.

Step by Step

One-Handed 'Scoop' Technique

Sharps safety devices are your first line of defense against sharps injuries, but when these devices are not available or are not suited for a clinical situation, the one-handed scoop technique may be used. Because this work practice control keeps fingers away from sharp needle tips, it is safer than recapping a needle using two hands.

1 First, place the cap on a hard, flat surface; then move your hand away from the cap.

2 Next, with one hand, hold the syringe and use the needle to "scoop-up" the cap.

3 Finally, when the cap covers the needle tip completely, hold the needle at the base near the hub and use the other hand to secure the cap.

4 The needle is now securely recapped.

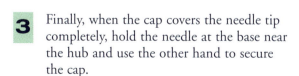
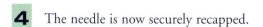
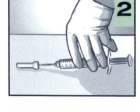
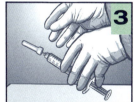
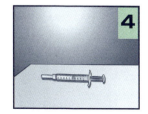

Safer Sharps Devices

Some sharps devices have safety features designed to reduce the risk of injury. An engineering control, some safety syringes incorporate a protective sheath that covers the needle to guard against injury.

Your practice setting should be examining devices with engineered safety features and using those that are found to be appropriate and effective for typical clinical situations.

Example of a Syringe with a Sharps Safety Feature

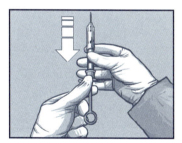

The sheath is pulled back to expose the needle for use.

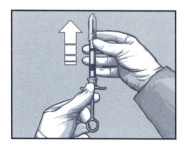

After use, the sheath is slid back to cover the needle.

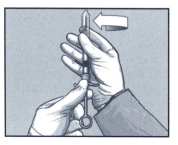

Some may lock in place.

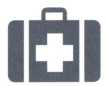

First Aid for Exposures

The first step in managing an exposure is always to perform basic first aid.

○ Clean wounds and skin sites with soap and water. In the case of a mucous membrane exposure, flush the affected area with cool water.

○ Do not use caustic agents on wounds. Never inject or apply bleach or other disinfectants to wound sites.

○ The use of an antiseptic is not contraindicated, but there is no evidence to suggest that using an antiseptic or squeezing the wound to express fluid reduces the risk of disease transmission.

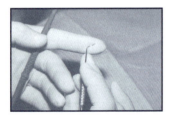

Patient care (exam) gloves can't protect against sharps injuries. In the event of an injury or other exposure, report the incident immediately so you can be referred for medical evaluation and follow-up. Some postexposure medications are available to reduce the risk of disease transmission, but these drugs must be given very soon (1-2 hours) after the exposure to be most effective.

Managing Exposures to Blood and Body Fluids

Although they are very effective when used routinely, infection control precautions cannot completely eliminate the risk of an exposure incident; accidents can happen. Exam and surgical gloves do not protect against sharps injuries, and unexpected spills and splashes of contaminated materials may expose eyes and other mucous membranes to possibly infectious materials.

Treat exposures as medical emergencies: Tend to them *immediately*. In case of an exposure to blood or other body fluids:

1 **Perform basic first aid to cleanse the wound or affected area.**

2 **Report the injury IMMEDIATELY to your employer or Infection Control Coordinator**. Provide as much information as you can about the incident (for example, the patient's bloodborne health status, if known; how and when the exposure happened; and your vaccination and response history). This information will help in evaluating and managing the exposure.

3 **Follow instructions for obtaining immediate and appropriate medical evaluation and follow-up care**. The physician or other qualified healthcare professional who handles your practice setting's occupational health program will evaluate your exposure and advise you of any options for medical management.

An exposure is a medical emergency. In the event of an exposure, report it immediately to your Infection Control Coordinator and follow instructions for receiving evaluation and follow-up care from your practice's designated healthcare professional.

An engineering control, free-standing needle recappers reduce the risk of sharps injuries by keeping fingers away from the sharp needle tip.

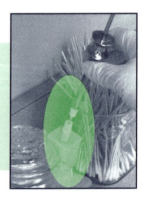

Flowchart for Management of Occupational Exposures to Bloodborne Pathogens

Before an Exposure Occurs...

Dental Health Care Personnel	Employer / Infection Control Coordinator	Qualified Healthcare Provider
○ Receives training in risks of occupational exposures, immediate reporting of injuries/exposures, and reporting procedures within the practice setting	○ Establishes referral arrangements and protocol for employees to follow in the event of exposures to blood or saliva via puncture injury, mucous membrane, or non-intact skin ○ Trains occupationally exposed employees in postexposure protocols ○ Makes available and pays for hepatitis B vaccine for workers at occupational risk	○ Contracts with dentist-employer to provide medical evaluation, counseling, and follow-up care to dental office employees exposed to blood or other potentially infectious materials ○ Keeps current on public health guidelines for managing occupational exposure incidents and is aware of evaluating healthcare provider's responsibilities ethically and by law

When an Exposure Incident Occurs...

Dental Health Care Personnel	Employer / Infection Control Coordinator	Qualified Healthcare Provider
1. Performs first aid 2. Reports injury to employer 3. Reports to the designated healthcare professional for medical evaluation and follow-up care, as indicated	1. Documents events in the practice setting 2. Immediately directs employee to evaluating healthcare professional 3. Sends to evaluating healthcare professional: ❑ copy of standard job description of employee ❑ exposure report ❑ source patient's identity and bloodborne infection status (if known) ❑ employee's HBV status and other relevant medical information ❑ copy of the Occupational Safety and Health Administration (OSHA) Bloodborne Pathogens Standard 4. Arranges for source patient testing, if the source patient is known and has consented 5. Pays for postexposure evaluation, and, if indicated, prophylaxis	1. Evaluates exposure incident, worker, and source patient for HBV, HCV, and HIV, maintaining confidentiality ❑ Arranges for collection and testing (with consent) of exposed worker and source patient as soon as feasible (if serostatus is not already known) ❑ In the event that consent is not obtained for HIV testing, arranges for blood sample to be preserved for up to 90 days (to allow time for the exposed worker to consent to HIV testing) ❑ Arranges for additional collection and testing as recommended by the U.S. Public Health Service/CDC ❑ Notifies worker of results of all testing and of the need for strict confidentiality with regard to source patient results ❑ Provides counseling ❑ Provides postexposure prophylaxis, if medically indicated 2. Assesses reported illnesses/side effects 3. Within 15 days of evaluation,
	6. Receives Written Opinion from evaluating healthcare professional ← ❑ Files copy of Written Opinion in employee's confidential medical record (if maintained by the dentist employer)	sends to the employer a Written Opinion, which contains (only):* ❑ documentation that the employee was informed of evaluation results and the need for any further follow-up
4. Receives copy of Written Opinion ←	❑ Provides copy of Written Opinion to exposed employee	❑ whether HBV vaccine was indicated and if it was received * All other findings or diagnoses remain confidential and are not included in the written report.

Sample Exposure Report / Questionnaire

Exposed Employee Information:

Name _____ Social Security No. _____ Job Title _____

Employer Name _____ Address _____

Time the injury occurred _____ Time reported _____ Date _____

Has the employee received hepatitis B vaccination?   ○ Yes   ○ No

If "Yes": Dates of vaccination   1. _____   2. _____   3. _____

Post-vaccination HBV antibody status, if known: _____ Positive _____ Titer   _____ Negative   _____ Unknown

Date of last Tetanus Vaccination: _____

Review of exposure incident follow-up procedures: ○ Yes   This form completed by _____

Exposure Incident Information:

Is the injury sharps related?   ○ Yes   ○ No

If "Yes,": Type of sharp _____ Brand _____

Work area where exposure occurred: _____

Procedure in progress: _____

How incident occurred: _____

Location of exposure (e.g., "right index finger"): _____

Did sharps involved have engineered injury protection?   ○ Yes   ○ No

    If "Yes":   Was the protective mechanism activated?   ○ Yes   ○ No

                The injury occurred (circle one) BEFORE / DURING / AFTER activation of protective mechanism.

    If "No":   In the employee's opinion, could a mechanism have prevented the injury: ○ Yes   ○ No

                If so, how? _____

In the employee's opinion, could any engineering, administrative, or work practice control have prevented the injury?   ○ Yes   ○ No

        Explain: _____

Source Patient Information:

Name _____ Chart No. _____

Telephone No. _____ Consent to release of information to evaluating healthcare professional   ○ Yes   ○ No

Patient's Signature _____

Review of source patient medical history: ○ Yes   ○ No

Verbally questioned regarding:

    History of Hepatitis B, Hepatitis C or HIV infection   ○ Yes   ○ No   If HIV-positive, antiretroviral medication history:

    High risk history associated with these diseases   ○ Yes   ○ No   _____

    Patient consents to be tested for HIV, HCV and HBV   ○ Yes   ○ No   _____

Evaluating Healthcare Professional Information:

Referred to (name of evaluating healthcare worker): _____

Questionnaire completed by: _____

Bill for fees to: _____

    Retain one copy in employee's confidential medical record; send one copy to evaluating healthcare professional with the exposed dental worker.

Common Questions and Answers

Is body fluid contact with intact skin an exposure?

No. Healthy, intact skin is a dental worker's best protective barrier. According to current CDC guidelines, follow-up is only required when the skin's integrity is compromised (for example, through chapping, abrasion, or an open wound) and the exposure involves blood, tissue, or other body fluids that are potentially infectious.

What if an injury occurs and we don't know who the source patient is?

If the exposure source is unknown — for example, for an injury that occurs while cleaning instruments from multiple operatories or more than one patient appointment — the circumstances of the exposure will be assessed by a qualified healthcare professional to determine the likelihood of HBV, HCV, or HIV transmission. Specific circumstances such as the type and severity of the exposure may suggest an increased or decreased risk of disease transmission, so postexposure treatment can be planned accordingly.

If we don't know who the source patient is, can we test the instrument that caused the injury?

Testing of needles or other sharp instruments implicated in an exposure is not recommended. This type of testing and analysis has not been proven to be reliable and could be hazardous to the lab personnel who would have to handle the contaminated sharp during serologic testing.

In the event of an exposure, can I go to my personal physician for evaluation and follow-up care?

In most cases, no. Family physicians or general practitioners may not be the best choice for assessing and managing occupational exposures. Evaluating healthcare professionals must be very familiar with current public health recommendations for managing exposures, antiretroviral therapy, and bloodborne disease transmission as well as the legal obligations and recordkeeping requirements. Your employer or Infection Control Coordinator should have identified a healthcare professional with the expertise in these matters. Often it is the same professional who manages vaccination schedules for the dental team.

Can medication after an exposure reduce the risk of disease transmission?

When indicated, postexposure prophylaxis should be started as soon as possible after exposure. Early administration affords the most benefit.

When warranted, HIV postexposure prophylaxis currently involves a four-week, three-drug (or more) regimen for all occupational exposures to HIV. The designated healthcare provider will assess the risks and make appropriate recommendations based upon current postexposure prophylaxis recommendations from Health Resources and Services Administration (HRSA)

There are currently no recommendations for postexposure prophylaxis against HCV. Because antiviral therapy may help when it is started early in the course of infection, testing for HCV is recommended in all exposure incidents. If HCV infection is identified, the employee should be referred to a specialist for medical management.

Did You Know...?

The exposure report helps the qualified healthcare professional determine if prophylaxis should be started and, if indicated, plan follow-up treatment.

Each exposure is evaluated individually for the likelihood that it will transmit a bloodborne disease like HBV, HCV, and HIV. Considerations include:

- the type and amount of body substance involved;
- the type of exposure (percutaneous injury, mucous membrane, or non-intact skin exposure);
- the infection status of the source; and
- the susceptibility of the exposed person.

The evaluating medical professional provides counseling on the risks of the exposure and on any options that may be available for reducing the risk of infection.

Of course, the best way to reduce risk of infection is to prevent exposure in the first place. Use engineering controls, work practice controls, personal protective equipment, and hand hygiene to minimize exposure risks.

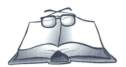

Recommended Readings and Resources

Centers for Disease Control and Prevention. Safer device implementation in health-care facilities. Available at: *www.cdc.gov/niosh/topics/bbp/safer/.*

American Dental Association. Employer Obligations After Exposure Incidents. Available at: *www.ada.org/en/science-research/osha-standard-of-occupational-exposure-to-bloodbor#Overview*

Kuhar DT, Henderson DK, Struble KA, et al. Updated U.S. Public Health Service guidelines for the management of occupational exposures to HIV and recommendations for postexposure prophylaxis. *Infection Control and Hospital Epidemiology* 2013;34(9):875-892. 2018 update available at: *stacks.cdc.gov/view/cdc/20711*

OSAP. The ABCs of Hepatitis. *Infection Control in Practice.* February 2007;6(7):1-2

Radcliffe RA, Bixler D, Moorman A, Hogan VA, Greenfield VS, Gaviria DM, Patel PR, Schaefer MK, Collins AS, Khudyakov YE, Drobeniuc J, Gooch BF, Cleveland JL. Hepatitis B virus transmissions associated with a portable dental clinic, West Virginia, 2009. *J Am Dent Assoc* 2013; 144(10): 1110–1118.

Redd JT, Baumbach J, Kohn W, Nainan O, Khristova M, Williams I. Patient-to-patient transmission of hepatitis B virus associated with oral surgery. *J Infect Dis* 2007;195(9):1311–1314.

Exercises in Understanding

1. Within your practice setting, to whom would you go to report an occupational exposure?

   Name: _____

   If this person is out to lunch, on vacation, or gone for the day, to whom would you report the injury?

   Name: _____

2. When giving multiple injections from the same syringe to one patient, how are needles recapped in your practice setting?

   ○ We use a needle recapper
   ○ We use the one-handed scoop technique

   If you use recappers, where are they located? _____
   _____

   If you use the one-handed scoop, have your Infection Control Coordinator watch you recap a needle and evaluate your technique.

3. What brands and types of sharps safety devices have been evaluated in your practice setting? _____
   _____

Self-Test

Before moving on, test yourself with some questions on the material.
(answers appear below)

1. Name three bloodborne pathogens.

   _____   _____   _____

2. The best protection against HBV infection is:
   a. engineering controls   c. vaccination
   b. safe work practices   d. personal protective equipment

3. True or False: I can identify all patients who are carrying a bloodborne disease by reading their medical histories.

4. The safest way to recap a needle that will be used for multiple injections on the same patient is:
   a. using your own two hands   c. holding the cap in your teeth
   b. having a coworker hold the cap   d. using a freestanding needle recapper
      while you insert the needle

5. The first step in managing an exposure is:
   a. report it to the appropriate person in the practice
   b. apply antiseptic
   c. cleanse or flush the exposure site
   d. postexposure prophylaxis

6. True or False: An occupational exposure is a medical emergency.

(1) Hepatitis B virus, hepatitis C virus, HIV (human immunodeficiency virus); (2) c; (3) False; (4) d; (5) c; (6) True.

Chapter 4

Hand Hygiene

Examining the Issues

Hand hygiene is the single most important way to prevent the spread of infection. Hand hygiene is an important part of standard precautions. Proper handwashing, hand antisepsis, or surgical hand antisepsis are simple acts that go a long way toward protecting you and your patients from infections.

Your skin is home to two groups of microorganisms: transient and resident.

○ Transient microorganisms are acquired through direct contact with patients or contaminated environmental surfaces. These microorganisms, which colonize the top layers of the skin and generally can be removed with routine handwashing, are most frequently associated with healthcare-acquired infections.

○ Resident flora attach to deeper layers of the skin. Although these microorganisms are harder to remove, they are less likely to be associated with healthcare-related infections and disease transmission.

In hospitals, lapses in hand hygiene have resulted in major disease outbreaks, many healthcare-associated infections, and the spread of antibiotic-resistant infections. Studies show that when hand hygiene improves, healthcare-associated infections decline.

In the dental setting, the risk of healthcare-acquired infection is much lower. Patients generally are not in urgent medical distress and more susceptible to infection. In addition, dental workers wear gloves for every patient care procedure.

Even though personal protective equipment is the norm for all direct patient-care activities, gloving is not a substitute for clean hands. For routine examinations and non-surgical procedures, perform hand hygiene by handwashing with either plain or antimicrobial soap or by using an alcohol-based handrub. You should also perform hand hygiene any time your skin comes in contact with contaminated materials. Alcohol-based handrubs are effective for hand hygiene, however, they should not be used when hands are visibly dirty.

Before surgical procedures, use a more rigorous hand-hygiene procedure with an antimicrobial product (described on p. 26).

The Bottom Line

Hand hygiene is considered the single most important way to reduce the risk of disease transmission. To ensure you always use the proper technique, consider the type and length of the procedures you'll be performing, the degree of contamination you're likely to encounter, and the persistence of antimicrobial activity you'll need.

> *Clean hands are the most important defense against spreading infection.*

Terms You Should Know

Alcohol-based hand rub

Antiseptic handwash

Antiseptic hand rub

Contaminated / contamination

Hand antisepsis

Hand hygiene

Handwashing

Healthcare-associated infection

Persistent activity

Plain soap

Resident Flora

Substantivity

Surgical hand antisepsis

Surgical hand scrub

Transient flora

Visibly soiled

Waterless antiseptic agent

For definitions, see "Glossary," beginning on page 166

Choosing Products for Hand Hygiene

When choosing hand hygiene products, keep in mind the following considerations:

○ **Broad-spectrum, persistent activity**
   For antimicrobial products, look for activity that continues after the handwash or hand rub.

○ **Low irritancy**
   To protect skin, consider a hand cleaner/antiseptic with skin softeners.

○ **Staff acceptance**
   Make sure hand hygiene products are accepted and used routinely. People may avoid using products they don't like.

○ **Potential allergies**
   Avoid ingredients that dental team members are allergic to. Chronic allergies can cause skin to crack and weep, which provides a portal of entry for microorganisms.

○ **Skin integrity after repeated use**
   Use compatible creams or lotions at the end of the work day to keep skin moist and healthy.

○ **Scent**
   An offensive odor can discourage routine use.

○ **Delivery system**
   Are sinks available? Can dispensers become contaminated?

○ **Cost per use**
   Look beyond the purchase price: Ineffective or unused products are no value.

Hand Hygiene in Practice

The type of hand hygiene technique you use depends on the type of procedure you'll be performing, the expected degree of contamination, and the desired persistence of antimicrobial action on the skin.

When hand hygiene is necessary	What agent to use
If hands are visibly dirty or contaminated, or when they are visibly soiled with blood or other body fluids...	○ ...wash hands with either a non-antimicrobial soap and water or an antimicrobial soap and water
If hands are not visibly soiled (for example, before putting on or after removing gloves) ...	○ ... wash hands with plain soap or an antimicrobial soap and water — or — ○ ... use an alcohol-based hand rub
Before surgery...	○ ... perform surgical hand antisepsis (described on p. 26) using either an antimicrobial soap or an alcohol-based hand rub with persistent activity

Always perform hand hygiene...

—upon entering clinic or radiography

○ ...when hands are visibly soiled.

○ ...before leaving the operatory or lab.

○ ...before and after treating any patient.

○ ...after touching objects with bare hands that may be contaminated with blood, saliva, or respiratory secretions.

○ ...before donning gloves.

○ ...after removing gloves.

○ ...after using the restroom.

○ ...before eating.

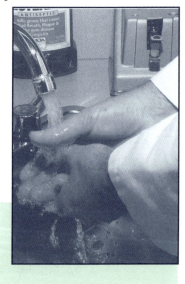

Gloving is NOT a substitute for handwashing.

To Wash or To Rub?

The pros and cons of different hand-hygiene techniques.

	(+)	**(-)**
Handwashing	❍ Can use plain or antimicrobial soap ❍ Effective antimicrobial activity with antiseptic soaps ❍ Effectiveness only minimally affected by organic matter ❍ Sinks readily available and accessible in most dental settings ❍ Familiar technique ❍ Allergic reactions to antimicrobial active ingredients are rare ❍ Regular use of hand lotions or creams prevents or treats handwashing-related, non-allergic skin irritation	❍ Frequent handwashing may cause skin dryness, chapping, and irritation ❍ Compliance with handwashing recommendations among hospital personnel is traditionally low ❍ More time-consuming than antiseptic hand rub ❍ Requires a sink and water ❍ Formulations with strong fragrances may be poorly tolerated by people with respiratory allergies

	(+)	**(-)**
Alcohol (Antiseptic) Hand Rub	❍ Provides more effective antiseptic action on visibly clean hands ❍ Faster hand asepsis than traditional handwashing ❍ Compared with routine handwashing, lower incidence of dryness and skin irritation when products containing skin softeners are regularly used ❍ Useful when sinks are not readily available or during boil-water notices (see p. 79) ❍ Allergic reactions to alcohol or additives are rare	❍ Not for use when hands are visibly dirty or contaminated ❍ Dispensing proper amount is critical ❍ Hands must be dry before agent is applied ❍ Frequent use can cause drying unless formulation contains emollients or other skin-conditioning agents ❍ Causes temporary stinging sensation upon application to broken skin ❍ Formulations with strong fragrances may be poorly tolerated by people with respiratory allergies ❍ Flammable; should be stored away from high temperatures or flames ❍ Some rubs can combine with residual glove powder on the hands, creating a gritty feeling ❍ Accessible handwashing stations are still required for use when an antiseptic hand rub is inappropriate

Did You Know....

The act of handwashing is actually more important than the type of soap you use. Each part of the handwashing process is necessary for removing microorganisms.

❍ **Lathering** pulls microorganisms away from the skin's crevices and suspends them.

❍ **Rinsing** washes them off your hands.

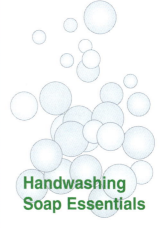

Handwashing Soap Essentials

For routine, nonsurgical handwashing in the dental setting:

❍ Use an amount of soap recommended by the manufacturer.

❍ No-touch soap dispensers are more hygienic.

Step-by-Step
Handwashing Technique

For handwashing with antimicrobial and non-antimicrobial soap:

1 Wet hands first with water.

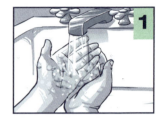

2 Apply plain or antimicrobial soap to hands and rub hands together to create a lather.

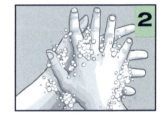

3 Rub hands together vigorously for at least 15 seconds, covering all surfaces of the hands and fingers.
  ○ **TIP**: Singing "Happy Birthday" to yourself while lathering is a good way to ensure you've washed for enough time.

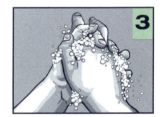

4 Rinse hands with water.
  ○ **TIP**: Avoid using hot water. Repeated exposure to hot water may increase the risk of dermatitis.

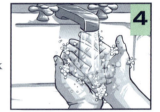

5 Dry hands thoroughly with a disposable towel.
  ○ **TIP**: Avoid using multiple-use cloth towels of the hanging or roll type.

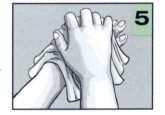

6 If the faucet is manual, use the towel to turn off the faucet so you don't recontaminate your hands.

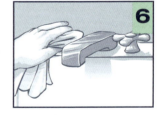

Step-by-Step

Alcohol Hand Rub Technique

When decontaminating hands with an alcohol-based hand rub:

1 Read and follow the manufacturer's recommendations for how much product to use.

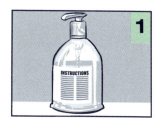

2 Apply product to palm of one hand and rub hands together, covering all surfaces of hands and fingers.

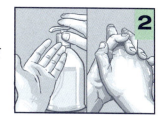

3 Continue rubbing hands together, covering all surfaces of the hands and fingers until the hands are dry.
○ **NOTE**: If hands feel dry after just 10-15 seconds of rubbing, you likely have used too little product.

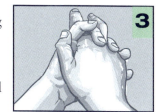

Common Questions and Answers

Can I wear acrylic fingernails at work?
Wearing artificial fingernails can compromise handwashing efforts; healthcare workers who wear artificial fingernails have been linked to serious disease outbreaks in high-risk hospital settings. Artificial nails also can make donning gloves more difficult and can cause tears more easily. As such, artificial nails are not recommended for workers in dental settings.

What about jewelry? Can I wear my engagement ring under my gloves?
Bacterial counts on hands are higher when rings are worn, so hand and arm jewelry should not be worn during surgical procedures. While rings do not seem to interfere with handwashing, they can make donning gloves more difficult and increase the risk of glove tears.

During non-surgical procedures, avoid any hand or nail jewelry that makes donning gloves more difficult or compromises the fit and integrity of the glove.

Can alcohol hand rubs take the place of handwashing?
Because alcohol-based hand rubs cannot be used on dirty hands, these products may never fully replace the need for handwashing in the traditional dental setting. When hands are not visibly dirty, alcohol-based hand rubs can be used to decontaminate hands. However, the alcohol rub must be applied to all surfaces of the hands and fingers and in the proper amount, following the manufacturer's instructions.

Tips and Advice for Hand Hygiene

To ensure effective hand hygiene in your practice setting:

○ Always read and heed manufacturers' instructions and warnings for using and storing hand-hygiene and skincare products.

○ Avoid using multiple-use, hanging- or roll-type cloth towels in healthcare settings. Disposable towels are more hygienic.

○ Do not add soap to a partially empty liquid soap dispenser. Repeated use of a soap dispenser may contaminate the container and soap inside. "Topping off" a partially empty dispenser may then cause contamination of the newly added soap. CDC recommends using disposable soap containers or washing and drying soap dispensers before refilling.

○ If alcohol hand rubs are used, place dispensers away from sinks to prevent any confusion between soap and the waterless alcohol formulations.

○ Keep nail tips short. Artificial nails have been implicated in microorganism and disease transmission from workers to patients.

More on the next page...

More Tips and Advice...

To ensure healthy skin and effective handwashing in your practice setting:

❍ Use hand lotions or creams to minimize adverse skin conditions associated with hand antisepsis or handwashing. Get information from manufacturers on the effects that lotions, creams, or alcohol-based hand antiseptics may have on the persistent effects of antimicrobial soaps or on gloves.

❍ During the clinic day, avoid using lotions that contain petroleum or have other oil-based ingredients. The agents may weaken glove material.

❍ Washing hands with soap and water after each use of an alcohol-based hand rub is not necessary and not recommended.

❍ Consider handwashing after 8-10 alcohol hand rubs to remove accumulated debris.

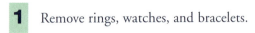

Step by Step

Surgical Hand Antisepsis Techniques

Before performing surgical procedures:

1 Remove rings, watches, and bracelets.

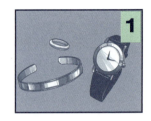

2 Use a nail cleaner under running water to remove debris from under fingernails.

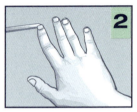

3 As described below, perform surgical hand antisepsis using either an antimicrobial soap or an alcohol-based hand rub with persistent activity.

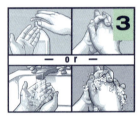

When using an antimicrobial soap:

Scrub hands and forearms for the length of time recommended by the manufacturer (usually 2-6 min.).
❍ **NOTE**: Long scrub times (e.g., 10 min.) are not necessary.

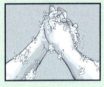

Dry thoroughly before donning sterile surgical gloves.

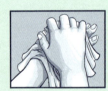

When using an alcohol-based surgical hand rub:

4 Follow the manufacturer's instructions.

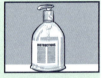

5 Before applying the alcohol solution, prewash hands and forearms with a non-antimicrobial soap and dry hands and forearms completely.

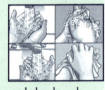

6 After applying the alcohol-based product as recommended, allow hands and forearms to dry thoroughly before donning sterile surgical gloves.

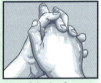

FDA Final Rule: Over-the-Counter Topical Antiseptics

The U.S. Food and Drug Administration (FDA) has issued a final rule determining that certain active ingredients in over-the-counter topical antiseptics used in health care settings are not considered generally recognized as safe and effective due to insufficient data. As part of the FDA's ongoing review of topical antiseptic active ingredients used in nonprescription antiseptic drug products, the FDA has issued a final rule determining that triclosan and 23 other active ingredients are not generally recognized as safe and effective used in certain over-the-counter (OTC) health care antiseptic products because no additional safety and effectiveness data for these active ingredients were provided to the agency. Because these ingredients are not used in the majority of currently marketed OTC health care antiseptic products, the agency expects little change to currently available products. The FDA has deferred for one year rulemaking on six active ingredients (benzalkonium chloride, benzethonium chloride, chloroxylenol, ethyl alcohol, isopropyl alcohol, and povidone-iodine) that are the most commonly used in OTC health care antiseptic products to provide manufacturers more time to complete the scientific studies necessary to fill the data gaps identified so that the agency can make a safety and efficacy determination about these ingredients. While we await the data on these commonly used active ingredients, the FDA recommends that health care personnel continue to use currently available products, consistent with infection control guidelines.

www.fda.gov/drugs/information-drug-class/qa-health-care-professionals-health-care-antiseptics

www.federalregister.gov/documents/2017/12/20/2017-27317/safety-and-effectiveness-of-health-care-antiseptics-topical-antimicrobial-drug-products-for

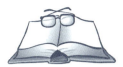

Recommended Readings and Resources

American Dental Association. Hand Hygiene for the Dental Team. *ADA Professional Product Review. 11 May 2015.* Available at: *www.ada.org/en/ publications/ada-profes- sional-product-review- ppr/archives/2015/vol_10 _iss_2/hand-hygiene-for- the-dental-team*

Centers for Disease Control and Prevention. Guideline for hand hy- giene in health-care set- tings: recommendations of the Healthcare Infec- tion Control Practices Advisory Committee and the HICPAC/ SHEA/APIC/IDSA Hand Hygiene Task Force. *Morbid Mortal Weekly Report* 2002; 51(RR16);1-44. Avail- able at: */www. cdc.gov/mmwr/preview/ mmwrhtml/rr5116a1.htm.*

Centers for Disease Control and Prevention. Hand Hygiene in Healthcare Settings. Available at: *www.cdc.gov/handhy- giene/*

Exercises in Understanding

1. What products and techniques do you use for hand hygiene ...
   ... when your hands are dirty? _____
   ... before gloving? _____
   ... after removing your gloves? _____

2. Have your Infection Control Coordinator evaluate your handwashing technique. Did you...

   ○ ... clean your fingertips and your thumbs?
   ○ ... scrub between each finger?
   ○ ... rinse and dry thoroughly to minimize skin irritation and chapping?

Self-Test

Before moving on, test yourself with some questions on the material.
(answers appear below)

1. List three desirable characteristics in a hand-hygiene product.

   _____   _____   _____

2. When hands are visibly soiled or contaminated, what types of hand hy- giene techniques are acceptable?
   a. handwash with plain soap and water   c. alcohol hand rub
   b. handwash with an antimicrobial soap and water   d. either a or b

3. True or False: When washing hands before surgery, you must use an an- timicrobial soap and scrub for at least 10 minutes.

4. What type of microorganisms found on the hands is more likely to be associated with disease transmission?
   a. resident flora   c. both are equally likely to transmit disease
   b. transient flora   d. neither can transmit disease

5. When selecting hand hygiene products, which of the following is not an important consideration?
   a. persistent effect   b. low irritancy   c. staff acceptance   d. color

(1) Low irritancy, accepted by staff, maintains skin integrity, pleasant scent, low cost per use, and (if antimicrobial) broad- spectrum, persistent antimicrobial activity; (2) d; (3) False; (4) b; (5) d.

Notes

Chapter 5

Personal Protective Equipment

Examining the Issues

As part of standard precautions, dental workers who are at risk of exposure to potentially infectious materials must wear personal protective equipment (PPE). Personal protective equipment includes gloves, masks, protective eyewear, face shields, and gowns or clinic jackets. PPE prevents exposure by providing a barrier between the patient's blood and body fluids and your skin, eyes, nose, and mouth. Employers are responsible for providing sufficient and appropriate personal protective equipment for all dental workers and must ensure that PPE is available and accessible to workers at all times.

Types of PPE routinely used in the dental setting include:

○ **Protective eyewear** (such as safety glasses or a chin-length face shield) to guard the eyes against exposure to droplet spatter and particulate debris.

○ **Surgical masks** to protect the mucous membranes of the nose and mouth against exposure to large droplets. Surgical masks do not keep you from inhaling aerosols.

○ **Protective apparel** to prevent contamination of clothing and protect your skin from blood and body fluid contamination.

○ **Medical gloves** — both patient examination and sterile surgical gloves — to protect your hands when you touch mucous membranes, blood, and other body fluids, or items contaminated with these materials. Wearing gloves also reduces the likelihood of transmitting microorganisms from your hands to patients during dental care procedures.

○ **Chemical- and puncture-resistant utility gloves** to protect your hands, wrists, and forearms during instrument processing and operatory clean-up procedures.

Choose personal protective equipment that is appropriate for the task at hand. For example, if you are going to be performing ultrasonic scaling, which not only puts you in contact with the patient's oral tissues but also creates lots of spatter, be sure to don gloves, face and eye protection, and protective apparel. If you are doing a brief oral soft-tissue exam, you may only need to wear medical gloves.

Terms You Should Know

Aerosols

Contaminated / contamination

Disinfectant

   Intermediate-level disinfectant

   Low-level disinfectant

Droplets / spatter

Face shield

Gloves

Mask

Medical gloves

Protective apparel

Protective eyewear

Utility gloves

Wicking

For definitions, see "Glossary," beginning on p. 166

The Bottom Line

Personal protective equipment can be very effective in preventing exposures to blood and other body fluids when routinely used in combination with engineering controls and safe work practices.

Choosing Face Protection

Consider the following to help you make the right choices for face protection in your practice setting.

Masks

○ **Sizing and fit**. Should fit the face well, creating a light seal over the nose and mouth; a form-fit over the bridge of the nose minimizes eyewear fogging.

○ **Comfort**. A comfortable fit encourages compliance.

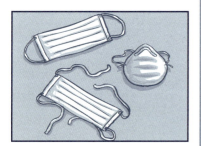

Surgical masks are available in cloth or cone styles, with earloops or tie backs.

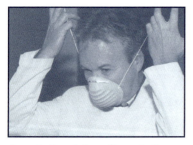

A surgical mask loses its protective qualities when it is wet. Change your mask whenever it becomes wet either from the outside (spatter) or the inside (condensation from your breath).

Preventing Exposure with PPE

Properly and routinely used, PPE can be very effective in preventing exposures to blood and other body fluids.

For all PPE...

○ Cover personal clothing and skin likely to be soiled with blood, saliva or other potentially infectious material.

○ Remove all personal protective barriers, including gloves, masks, eyewear, and gowns, before leaving work areas like operatories, the lab, and the instrument processing area.

○ Never wear PPE to the breakroom, restroom, or out of the dental setting.

○ Hand hygiene is always the last step after removing and disposing of PPE.

Face Protection

Face protection includes masks, protective eyewear, and chin-length face shields that protect the mucous membranes of the eyes, nose, and mouth.

○ When a procedure is expected to create splash or spatter of blood, body fluids, or materials contaminated with these fluids, wear a surgical mask and eye protection with solid side shields.

❏ Safety glasses or goggles and a surgical mask can be used for procedures where small amounts of spatter or splashes are likely. A face shield with surgical mask may be useful when more protection is needed.

○ Protective eyewear may be provided to patients to shield their eyes from spatter or debris generated during treatment.

○ Decontaminate reusable eye and face protection (protective eyewear, face shields) between patients.

❏ Use soap and water for eyewear and face shields that are not contaminated with blood.

❏ Use an intermediate-level disinfectant for protective equipment that shows visible blood. (For more on disinfectant categories and choices, see Ch. 8, Environmental Infection Control.)

○ Change masks between patients, or during patient treatment if the mask becomes wet.

Protective Apparel

Protective apparel covers your skin, street clothes, or uniform, preventing their contamination. Suitable choices include reusable or disposable gowns or laboratory coats with high necks.

○ Wear long-sleeved protective clothing when skin or clothing is likely to be soiled.

❏ Street clothes or uniforms, pants, and shirts that are not intended to protect against a hazard are *not* personal protective equipment.

○ Change protective apparel when it becomes visibly soiled.

○ Change protective apparel immediately or as soon as possible if it is penetrated by blood or body fluids.

(a) A surgical mask and safety glasses with solid side shields protects mucous membranes of the eyes, nose, and mouth; (b) Providing patients with safety glasses protects their eyes from debris generated during treatment procedures.

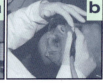

Gloves

○ Wear examination gloves when there is a potential for contacting blood or body fluids, mucous membranes, non-intact skin or potentially infectious material.

○ Wear a new pair of examination gloves for each patient, remove them promptly after use, and wash hands immediately to avoid transfer of microorganisms to other patients or environments.

○ Remove gloves that are torn, cut, or punctured as soon as safety permits. Wash hands before regloving.

○ Never wash surgical or patient examination gloves before use. Never wash, disinfect, or sterilize gloves for reuse. Doing so may compromise the material and increase the flow of liquid through undetected holes ("wicking").

○ Wear sterile surgeon's gloves when performing oral surgical procedures. In the U.S., sterile surgical gloves must meet quality-control standards for sterility established by the Food and Drug Administration.

○ Use puncture- and chemical-resistant heavy-duty utility gloves for cleaning instruments, performing decontamination, and during housekeeping procedures that involve potential blood or body fluid contact.

○ Ensure that task-specific gloves are readily accessible in the appropriate sizes and materials.

❏ Stock gloves made of alternative materials for dental workers and patients who may be allergic to latex proteins or other glove components. Glove-associated allergies are discussed in Ch. 6, Contact Dermatitis and Latex Allergy.

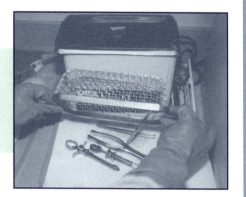

Puncture-resistant utility gloves protect against sharps injuries during instrument processing.

Choosing Eye Protection

Look for the following features in the eye protection used in your dental work setting.

Eyewear / face shields

○ **Impact resistance.** Look for impact-resistant plastic

○ **Side protection.** Coverage around the eyes

○ **Suited for specific applications in practice.**

❏ For large amounts of spatter / debris, chin-length full-face shields may be more comfortable and effective; added coverage helps keep masks dry

Personal eyewear is not recommended for eye protection

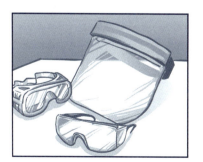

In combination with a mask, goggles, face shields, and safety glasses with side shields provide protection from mucous membrane exposures.

Types of Gloves Used In Dentistry

Glove type	Used for...
Patient examination gloves	Patient care, examinations, and other nonsurgical procedures involving contact with mucous membranes
Sterile surgical gloves	Oral surgical procedures
Heavy Duty Utility	Housekeeping procedures (e.g., cleaning and disinfection)
	Handling contaminated sharps or chemicals
	Not for use during patient care

Choosing Gloves

The dental marketplace is full of options for personal protective equipment. Consider the following to help you make the right glove choices for your practice setting.

Patient-Care Gloves

❍ **Sizes**. Stock sizes to fit all at-risk workers.
❍ **Fit**. Look for a snug, comfortable fit; not too tight or loose.
❍ **Allergies and sensitivities**. Provide non-latex gloves for latex-allergic workers and patients; low-total-protein or low-allergen latex gloves may lower the risk of developing an allergy.
❍ **Ambidextrous vs. hand-specific**. Less expensive ambidextrous gloves may contribute to fatigue and repetitive stress disorders; more expensive hand-specific gloves offer better fit, more comfort, and less hand and wrist strain.
❍ **Shelf life**. Affected by temperature, humidity, or light.

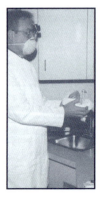

When ready to begin treatment, wash and thoroughly dry your hands, then put on fresh gloves. Protective clothing, a new mask, and clean eyewear should already be in place.

Utility Gloves

❍ **Puncture-resistance**. To protect against injury.

Donning PPE

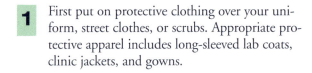

Don patient-care PPE in the reverse order of what you change the most during the course of the clinic day. Gloves are changed most often, face protection less often, and clothing least often of all.

1 First put on protective clothing over your uniform, street clothes, or scrubs. Appropriate protective apparel includes long-sleeved lab coats, clinic jackets, and gowns.

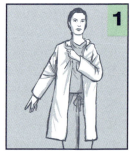

2 Put on a surgical mask.

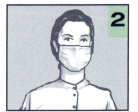

3 Add protective eyewear (for example, safety glasses with side shields, goggles, or a face shield).

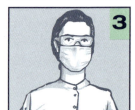

4 When you are ready to begin the procedure, wash and thoroughly dry your hands.
NOTE: When hands are not visibly soiled, an alcohol-based hand rub may be used instead of handwashing.

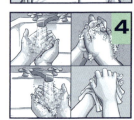

5 Holding one glove at the cuff, place the opposite hand inside the glove and pull it onto the hand. Adjust for fit. Repeat with a new glove on the other hand.

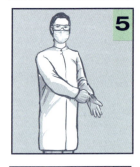

6 You are now ready to begin patient care.

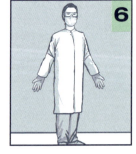

Removing PPE

Use care when removing personal protective equipment to prevent contaminating hands, clothing, skin, and mucous membranes.

Gloves

Change gloves between patients and as needed if you must respond to treatment interruptions. To remove exam gloves:

1 Use your gloved hand to grab the other glove at the outside cuff. Pull downward, turning the glove inside-out as it pulls away from your hand.

2 For the other hand, use your ungloved fingers to grab the inside (uncontaminated area) of the cuff of the remaining glove. Pull downward to remove the glove, turning it inside out.

3 Wash and thoroughly dry hands before regloving.
NOTE: If no visible contamination exists and gloves have not been torn or punctured during use, an antiseptic hand rub may be used in place of handwashing. Handwashing and rinsing may be preferred if hands are damp with perspiration or to remove glove powder and chemicals.

Masks

Change masks between patients or when they become damp from external contamination or from condensation of moist, exhaled air. (Practical experience suggests about every 20 min.)

! Remove mask using ungloved hands. Contact only the mask's ties or elastic strap.

Eyewear

Clean reusable eye and face protection between patients.

1 Remove protective eyewear by touching the ear rests, head band, or clips . Place them on a disposable towel out of the way.

2 If contaminated with blood, put on gloves and disinfect according to the manufacturer's instructions; if not, wash with soap and water.

Apparel

To remove visibly soiled clothing:

1 Fold the soiled area away from the body to remove. Be careful not to contaminate your hands.

2 Discard disposable garments or place reusable protective apparel into the designated container for contaminated laundry.

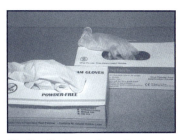

Stock patient care gloves in sizes to fit all dental workers. Also, consider allergies and sensitivities.

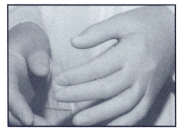

Look for a comfortable fit in patient care gloves. They should be neither too tight nor too loose.

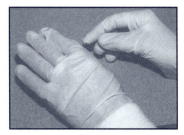

Gloves that are too loose can compromise tactility and control.

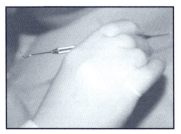

Gloves that are too tight exert pressure on the hands, possibly contributing to muscle strain and injury.

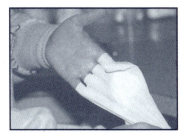

Only touch the inside (clean side) of a contaminated glove with your bare hand. Turn the cuff inside out and pull gently to remove.

The Right PPE for the Purpose

The personal protective equipment you use for any given task should protect you against any hazards to which you otherwise would be exposed.

Personal Protective Equipment

Suggested PPE for Tasks within the Dental Setting

Task	Gloves (patient examination or sterile surgical)	Face Protection (e.g., mask, face shield)	Eye Protection (e.g., safety glasses, face shield)	Garment (e.g., lab coat, gown, clinic jacket)	Utility Gloves	Other* (below)	Comment* (below) None
Patient care							
Greeting the patient in the reception area							X
Taking a medical history			1*				X
Performing an oral exam	X	3*	3*	1*			
Polishing teeth	X	X	X	X			
Scaling (manual)	X	X	X	X			
Scaling (ultrasonic)	X	X	X	X			
Suctioning during a cavity preparation	X	X	X	X			
In-operatory charting				1*		2*	X
Taking an impression	X	3*	3*	1*			
Answering the telephone during treatment						2*	X
Instrument processing							
Placing instruments in a holding solution (to keep them moist until they can be cleaned)		X	X	X	X		
Loading the ultrasonic cleaner / instrument washer		X	X	X	X		
Handscrubbing instruments		X	X	X	X		
Wrapping instruments for sterilization				1*	X		
Loading the sterilizer				1*	X		
Removing instrument packs from the sterilizer						4*	
Distributing/storing wrapped, sterile instrument packets							X
Operatory clean-up							
Transporting instruments from operatory to reprocessing area	X			1*			
Environmental surface disinfection (using spray-wipe-spray technique)		X	X	X	X		
Placing a clean surface barrier on an uncontaminated surface				1*			X
Maintenance / quality control							
Cleaning the ultrasonic chamber, discarding and replacing solution		X	X	X	X		
Recording results of sterilizer monitoring							X

* Other / Comments:

(**1**) Although it may not be required, it is acceptable to leave on protective clothing that has been worn throughout patient treatment as long as it is not visibly soiled. Never wear personal protective equipment in break rooms, offices, or reception areas.

(**2**) Alternative to removing gloves, vinyl overgloves (foodhandlers' gloves) can be donned to limit the spread of contamination to clinical contact surfaces during treatment interruptions.

(**3**) Optional; may provide additional protection against non-bloodborne disease transmission.

(**4**) Heat-resistant gloves protect against burns from hot instrument packs.

Common Questions and Answers

When should I wear gloves?

Wear gloves whenever you put your hands into any patient's mouth or touch instruments, equipment, or surfaces that may be contaminated with blood or body fluids. Always use a new pair of gloves for every patient.

What type of gloves should I wear?

The type of gloves you should wear depends on what tasks you are performing. Three type of gloves are available:
- ○ **Disposable patient examination gloves** for procedures involving contact with oral mucous membranes. These gloves can be made of latex, vinyl, nitrile, polyurethane, and other materials.
- ○ **Sterile disposable gloves (surgical gloves)** for use when sterility is necessary such as during oral surgical procedures.
- ○ **Chemical-resistant, puncture-resistant utility gloves** for use when cleaning instruments, equipment, and contaminated surfaces. As long as they are puncture-resistant, rubber household gloves may be used.

Can gloves be washed and reused?

Never reuse surgical or patient examination gloves. Washing these gloves may damage them and cause "wicking," which increases the flow of liquid through undetected holes in the gloves.

If they are not punctured or torn, utility gloves may be reused, but they should be properly decontaminated before reuse (more info in Ch. 7, Sterilization and Disinfection of Patient Care Items).

What if my glove tears?

If your gloves become torn, cut, or punctured, remove them immediately and dispose of them properly. Wash your hands thoroughly with soap and water, dry them well, and put on a new pair of gloves before resuming patient care.

If I wear a face shield, must I wear a mask underneath?

Yes, face shields require the use of a surgical mask as well. Surgical masks protect the patient from healthcare worker secretions; a face shield alone doesn't offer such protection, nor does it prevent workers from drawing in mists from handpieces and ultrasonic scalers.

How should we dispose of contaminated patient care gloves?

Contaminated patient care gloves do not qualify as regulated waste. Dispose of them with other non-regulated contaminated waste (such as masks, patient bibs, and disposable air-water syringe tips) in the regular office trash unless your state or local law requires special handling.

Do I need to change my lab coat between patients?

Unless your coat is visibly soiled or penetrated by blood or body fluids, there is no need to put on a fresh coat for each patient.

Can I take my lab coat home with me to launder?

In the United States, dental workers are not allowed to take their personal protective equipment home to launder. Laundering of PPE is the responsibility of the employer.

Choosing Protective Clothing

Looking for the right protective garments? Try the following desirable features on for size:

Protective Garments

- ○ **Barrier to contaminants**. The garment should protect skin and street clothes that could become contaminated.
- ○ **Appropriate for each task**. In the context of each procedure routinely performed in the practice, consider:
  - ❑ Protection. From splash, spatter, and debris.
  - ❑ Comfort. Fabrics that "breathe."
- ○ **Design and features**.
  - ❑ High-necked/high-collared.
  - ❑ Long sleeves.
  - ❑ Covers the knees when seated (if performing sit-down dentistry).
- ○ **Cost-effectiveness**. Compare costs of buying disposable garments in bulk; buying and installing a washer and dryer and staff time doing laundry; and using a medical laundry service.

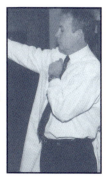

Lab coats, gowns, and clinic jackets protect street clothes, uniforms, and skin from contamination.

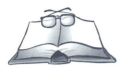

Recommended Readings and Resources

Centers for Disease Control and Prevention. "Laundry facilities and equipment." Guidelines for environmental infection control in health-care facilities: recommendations of CDC and the Healthcare Infection Control Practices Advisory Committee (HICPAC). *MMWR Morbid Mortal Weekly Report* 2003;52 (RR10). Available at *www.cdc.gov/mmwr//preview/mmwrhtml/rr5210a1.htm.*

Miller CH. Infection Control and Management of Hazardous Materials for the Dental Team, 6th edition St. Louis: Elsevier, 2018.

Molinari JA. Clinic jackets and gowns: a misunderstood personal protection equipment requirement? *Compend Contin Educ Dent. 2001;22:494.*

Did You Know... ?

A surgical mask loses its protective qualities when it gets wet.

When a mask gets wet, the material doesn't "breathe" as well as it should. This causes more airflow to pass by edges of the mask. It also may cause you to inhale harder, pulling the damp, contaminated mask closer to your nose and mouth.

Your surgical mask can become wet simply from your exhaling warm, moist air into it. Your breath condenses on the mask's surface, leaving it damp. The mask's outer surface also can become contaminated with droplets from spray and spatter or from touching the mask with contaminated fingers.

Always change your mask between patients or if possible, during patient treatment when it becomes wet from either the inside or the outside.

Remember: Masks are to be worn over your nose and mouth; they offer no protection when worn around your neck or on top of your head. Improperly worn, they can even spread contamination to your clothes, skin, and hair.

Exercises in Understanding

For your last patient appointment, did you...:

	Yes	No
.... wear disposable gloves?		
.... wash your hands before you gloved?		
... use a new pair of gloves just for this patient?		
... remove your gloves when treatment was complete and contaminated instruments had been removed?		
... wash your hands immediately after removing gloves?		
... wear chemical-resistant utility gloves while cleaning instruments and decontaminating equipment surfaces?		
... wear facial protection?		
... avoid touching the surface of your mask with contaminated gloves during treatment?		
... avoid touching your contaminated mask with bare hands after treatment?		
... clean and if necessary, disinfect your safety glasses or face shield after patient treatment?		
... protect yourself and your street clothes or uniform by wearing a gown, lab coat, or jacket?		

Count the number of "No" answers.

0-1 — You are using protective barriers effectively. Continue these practices with every patient.

2-3 — Your use of personal protective equipment was almost ideal with this patient. Try to have all your answers in the "Yes" column with the next patient.

4+ — You need to make better use of personal protective equipment. Read Ch. 2 and 3 of this book again and try to put more of the recommendations into practice.

Self-Test

Before moving on, test yourself with some questions on the material.
(answers appear below)

1. List three important features of a protective garment.
   _____ _____ _____

2. Before donning exam gloves, they should be:
   a. washed   b. disinfected   c. sterilized   d. none of the above

3. Laundering protective clothing is the responsibility of:
   a. the dental workers   c. the Centers for Disease Control and Prevention
   b. the employer   d. none of the above

4. Protective apparel must be removed:
   a. before leaving the work area   c. when penetrated by blood or saliva
   b. when visibly soiled   d. all of the above

5. Which of the following is not considered appropriate protective eyewear?
   a. goggles   c. standard prescription eyeglasses
   b. safety glasses   d. face shield

6. After patient treatment, hold your mask by the _____
   to remove it with ungloved hands.
   a. ties or elastic strap   c. underside, where it rests against the skin
   b. body   d. any of the above

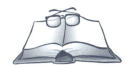

Recommended Readings and Resources

OSAP. If Saliva Were Red: A Visual Lesson on Infection Control. *www.osap.org*

Palenik CJ. Personal protective equipment. *Dent Econ* 2003;93(2):72.

Palenik CJ. The eyes have it. *RDH* 2003;23(2):69.

Rawson D. The basics of surgical mask selection. *Infect Control Today* 2003;7(3):32.

Shulman ER, Brehm WT. Dental clinical attire and infection-control procedures. *JADA* 2001;132:508.

Centers for Disease Control and Prevention. Healthcare Associated Infections (HAI). Protecting Healthcare Personnel. Available at: *www.cdc.gov/HAI/prevent/ppe.html*

OSHA. Standard Interpretations. Compliance with OSHA Bloodborne Pathogen Standard. 02 Feb 2009. (includes discussion of laundering PPE). Available at: *www.osha.gov/pls/oshaweb/owadisp.show_document?p_table=INTERPRETATIONS&p_id=27008*

(1) Long-sleeves, high neck or collar, covers the knees when you are seated if you perform sit-down dentistry; (2) d; (3) b; (4) d; (5) c; (6) a.

Notes

Chapter 6

Contact Dermatitis and Latex Allergy

 ## Examining the Issues

While the benefits of gloving and handwashing can't be overstated, some adverse skin conditions can develop as a result of frequent and repeated handwashing, exposure to chemicals, and glove use.

Although adverse skin reactions occur frequently among dental workers, true latex allergy does not. Any glove-associated condition requires diagnosis by an allergist or dermatologist so that proper corrective actions can be taken.

○ **Irritant contact dermatitis** is very common among dental workers. Caused by physical irritation of the skin, it presents as dry, itchy, irritated areas of the skin around the area of contact with the offending agent. Irritant contact dermatitis is not an allergic reaction. Nonetheless, any condition that compromises healthy skin increases the risk of exposure to blood and other body fluids. (Remember: Cracks and breaks in the skin can provide a portal of entry for pathogens.)

○ **Allergic contact dermatitis** (also called type IV or delayed hypersensitivity) is a skin condition that can result from exposure to chemicals such as methacrylates (found in bonding agents), glutaraldehydes, ortho-phthalaldehyde, and rubber manufacturing chemicals. Allergic contact dermatitis often appears as a rash beginning several hours or even days after contact. Like irritant dermatitis, it usually is confined to the area of contact but can extend slightly beyond the contact area.

○ **Latex hypersensitivity** (also referred to as "latex allergy") is a potentially life-threatening allergy to the proteins contained in natural rubber latex, which is a common glove material. Also referred to as a type I immediate allergy, this is a more serious, whole-body allergic reaction that usually begins within minutes of exposure but also can occur hours later. Although symptoms can vary, they often affect the eyes, nose, and skin. More common reactions include runny nose, sneezing, itchy eyes, scratchy throat, hives, and itchy, burning skin sensations. More severe symptoms include asthma (marked by difficult breathing, coughing spells, and wheezing), cardiovascular and gastrointestinal symptoms, and in rare cases, anaphylaxis. In especially severe reactions that are not medically managed, a type I allergy can result in death.

Latex and glove chemicals are not the only allergens found in the dental office. Metals, plastics, chemicals, or other materials used in dental care also are common allergens. A thorough health history and appropriately avoiding contact with potential allergens will minimize the possibility of adverse reactions.

 ## The Bottom Line

Properly diagnosing occupational allergies and skin conditions is the key to successfully managing them. Because symptoms are often similar (especially for irritant and contact dermatitis), evaluation by an allergist or dermatologist is essential for determining the cause and the course of treatment for any suspected occupational allergies.

Whether patient or dental worker, latex-allergic individuals should avoid all contact with latex-containing products. Although this may be a challenge in some dental practices, several strategies can reduce exposure to allergens in the dental setting.

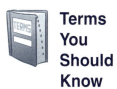 ## Terms You Should Know

Allergen

Allergic contact dermatitis

Anaphylaxis

Handwashing

Irritant contact dermatitis

Latex hypersensitivity

Natural rubber latex

Portal of entry

For definitions, see "Glossary," beginning on p. 166

Glove Powder and Latex Allergy

The Food and Drug Administration (FDA or Agency) has determined that Powdered Surgeon's Gloves, Powdered Patient Examination Gloves, and Absorbable Powder for Lubricating a Surgeon's Glove present an unreasonable and substantial risk of illness or injury and that the risk cannot be corrected or eliminated by labeling or a change in labeling. Consequently, FDA is banning these devices. www.federalregister.gov/documents/2016/12/19/2016-30382/banned-devices-powdered-surgeons-gloves-powdered-patient-examination-gloves-and-absorbable-powder

Latex-allergic workers should wear only non-latex gloves, for example, those made of nitrile or vinyl.

Preventing and Reducing Exposure to Latex Allergens

Because of the potentially serious consequences, you and your dental team members must look for and accommodate latex allergies in patients and among staff.

Education

○ Know the signs, symptoms, and diagnoses of skin reactions associated with frequent hand hygiene and glove use.

   ❑ If you think you have an occupational allergy, get evaluated, get a diagnosis, and let the diagnosis drive the decision on how to manage the problem in your work setting.

Patient Screening

○ Screen all patients for latex allergy. Take a thorough health history and consult with the patient's physician if necessary. Obtain a medical consultation when latex allergy is suspected.

   ❑ Ask about reactions to common household products that contain latex, like cleaning gloves, balloons, rubber bands, and elastics.

   ❑ Ask about common predisposing conditions: previous history of allergies; a history of spina bifida; urogenital anomalies; or allergies to avocados, kiwis, nuts, or bananas.

Managing Latex-Allergic Patients

○ Provide a "latex safe" environment.

   ❑ To treat the latex-allergic patient in the safest possible way, keep non-latex gloves and treatment kits stocked and use them on latex-allergic patients.

   ❑ Identify all latex-containing products and devices in the operatory to prevent their accidental introduction to the hypersensitive patient. Consider sources of latex other than gloves, for example, prophylaxis cups, rubber dams, orthodontic elastics, anesthetic carpules, and medication vials.

   ❑ Have emergency treatment kits with latex-free supplies available at all times.

   ❑ Be alert to the signs and symptoms of an allergic reaction and be prepared to treat complications should they arise.

   ❑ Frequently change ventilation filters and vacuum bags used in latex-contaminated areas.

   ❑ Use signs, verbal instruction, and checklists to prevent dental team members from bringing latex-containing materials into the treatment area.

   ❑ Remove all latex-containing products from the patient's vicinity. Adequately cover/isolate any latex-containing devices that cannot be removed from the treatment environment.

❏ Thoroughly wash your hands. In a highly latex-allergic patient, contact with someone who has worn latex gloves could trigger a reaction.

○ If possible, maintain a latex-safe treatment room. (In practices with open operatories, this option may not be feasible.)

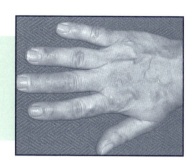

If you think you have occupational allergies, get evaluated, get a diagnosis, and let the diagnosis drive decisions on how to manage the problem.

Keeping Hands Healthy

As a dental worker, your hands are your greatest tools, and intact skin is your best barrier against infectious microorganisms.

When skin is irritated and inflamed, its natural barrier properties are compromised, making it more susceptible to penetration by potential allergens and pathogens. Also, inflamed skin contains high numbers of microorganisms, and handwashing will not remove bacteria from irritated skin. Non-intact (broken) skin also offers a portal of entry for bloodborne pathogens.

For the best protection your skin can provide, keep hands and skin healthy both inside and outside the dental setting.

○ Always rinse and dry hands thoroughly after handwashing.

○ Avoid bare-handed contact with sensitizers and irritants such as disinfectants, acrylic monomers, and antimicrobial and pharmacological solutions.

○ Be wary of chemicals that can permeate glove materials. Bonding agents, acrylics, and bases and liners should not be placed on or in contact with gloved hands. Wear chemical- and puncture resistant utility gloves when working with glutaraldehyde.

○ Use hand creams and lotions to prevent dryness and maintain skin integrity, but choose carefully to ensure compatibility between lotions, antiseptic products, and glove materials.

   ❏ Preparations containing petroleum and other oil-based ingredients may degrade some glove materials. Water-based lotions are typically a better choice. Oil-based skin softeners may be used at the end of the work day.

○ Outside of the dental setting, use protective gloves when mixing or handling household chemicals. Irritants in household products such as cleaning agents, glues, and solvents can worsen the effects of the soaps, gloves, and chemicals encountered during the work day.

○ Wear task-appropriate protective gloves when work around the house will be hard on the hands, for example, when gardening or performing car repairs.

○ Use a moisturizing agent after at-home handwashing to keep skin from becoming dry.

Eliminating Latex in the Dental Setting

To safely treat a latex allergic patient, you must identify all latex-containing products and devices in the operatory and prevent their accidental introduction to the hypersensitive patient.

While latex gloves may be an obvious product to avoid, consider other sources of latex.

Latex in dental settings

Anesthesia masks
Anesthetic carpules (stoppers)
Blood pressure cuffs
Catheters
Dental dams
Disposable gloves
Endotracheal tubes
Electrode pads
Gloves
Goggles
Injection ports
Intravenous tubing
Oral and nasal airways
Orthodontic bands
Respirators
Rubber aprons
Rubber tops of multi-dose vials
Stethoscopes
Surgical masks
Syringes
Tourniquets
Wound drains

Occupational Dermatitis and Latex Allergy

Condition	Cause	Symptoms	Corrective action
Irritant contact dermatitis	Physical irritation; not an allergy May be caused by unrinsed scrubs, soaps, disinfectants; excessive powder; occlusion; hyperhydration; excessive chemical additives	Acute: inflammation, burning, itching Chronic: dry, thickened skin; cracking; sores; spaced bumps Typically limited to areas of contact	Consult an allergist/dermatologist Use moisturizing lotions and creams during and after work (avoid products containing petroleum; they can degrade glove materials) Pay careful attention to handwashing techniques (especially rinsing)
Allergic contact dermatitis Delayed (type IV) hypersensitivity	Allergy to: Chemicals found in the dental practice setting, including methacrylates, glutaraldehyde, and chemicals used in the glove manufacturing process	Acute: small, clustered bumps; vesicles; itching; redness; pain Chronic: dry, thickened skin; cracking; sores; spaced bumps Redness, vesicle formation typically develops several hours after contact Usually confined to but may extend slightly beyond the area of contact	Consult an allergist/dermatologist; get a definitive diagnosis Select a glove that is low in the offending chemical allergen
Latex allergy Immediate (type I) hypersensitivity	Allergy to the proteins in natural rubber latex	Hives, swelling, watery eyes, runny nose, difficulty breathing, abdominal cramps, dizziness, low blood pressure, tachycardia (rapid heart rate), anaphylaxis	Requires immediate emergency care during acute reactions; prepare for an anaphylactic emergency Consult an allergist Ensure a powder-free environment: ☐ Use non-latex gloves and dental products; flag patient chart for latex-free care ☐ Asymptomatic healthcare workers at risk should wear only non-latex gloves

Common Questions and Answers

How do I know if I'm allergic to glove materials?

See an allergist or dermatologist for evaluation and diagnosis. A skin prick test or blood test can diagnose a latex type-I hypersensitivity. Patch testing, in which potential allergens are placed in contact with the skin for several days, will determine if you have any contact (type IV) allergies, including those to common glove chemicals.

My coworker has a documented allergy to latex. Do we all have to switch to latex-free products?

Many healthcare settings with latex-allergic workers have found that providing the affected worker with non-latex materials and switching the rest of the team to synthetic gloves or to low-allergen latex gloves was sufficient. The worker's allergist should be able to provide direction on creating a safe workplace.

Exercises in Understanding

1. Walk through your operatory looking for items containing latex. How many items containing latex can you find?

2. Find the latex-free treatment kit in your practice setting. Does it contain:

    _____ non-latex gloves in the right sizes for both doctor and staff?

    _____ synthetic rubber dam?

    _____ non-latex prophy cups?

    _____ anesthetic in a non-latex-containing delivery system?

    other _____

3. Where is your practice setting's latex-free medical emergency kit located? Is it easily accessible? When was it last updated?

    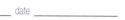
    _____ date _____

Self-Test

Before moving on, test yourself with some questions on the material.
(answers appear below)

1. Which of the following is not an allergic condition?
a. irritant contact dermatitis   b. allergic contact dermatitis   c. latex hypersensitivity

2. Hives are a symptom of which condition?
a. irritant contact dermatitis   b. allergic contact dermatitis   c. latex hypersensitivity

3. True or False: The US Food and Drug Administration (FDA) banned powdered surgical and examination gloves.

4. Name three latex-containing products typically used in your operatories.

_____   _____   _____

(1) a; (2) c; (3) True; (4) Examples include gloves, prophy cups, orthodontic bands, anesthetic carpule stoppers, medication vials, blood pressure cuffs, and rubber dam

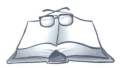

Recommended Readings and Resources

Hamann CP, Rodgers PA, Sullivan K. Allergic contact dermatitis in dental professionals: effective diagnosis and treatment. *JADA* 2003;134(2):185.

Hamann CP, Rodgers PA, Sullivan K. Management of dental patients with allergies to natural rubber latex. *Gen Dent* 2002; 50(6):526.

OSHA. Potential for Sensitization and Possible Allergic Reaction to Natural Rubber Latex Gloves and other Natural Rubber Products. 2008. Available at: *www.osha.gov/dts/shib/shib012808.pdf*

Schmid K, Christoph Broding H, Niklas D, Drexler H. Latex sensitization in dental students using powder-free gloves low in latex protein: a cross-sectional study. *Contact Dermatitis* 2002;47(2):103-8.

Notes

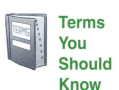

Chapter 7

Sterilization and Disinfection of Patient-Care Items

Patient-care items — that is, dental instruments, devices, and equipment — are categorized based on their risk of transmitting a disease. The degree of contact they have with patients suggests the risk of disease transmission they carry.

- **Critical items** penetrate soft tissue or bone. They have the greatest risk of transmitting infection and should always be sterilized using heat.
- **Semicritical items** touch only mucous membranes or nonintact skin. As such, they have a lower risk of transmission than critical items. In dentistry, the majority of semicritical items are heat-tolerant, therefore, they should also be sterilized using heat. If a semicritical item is heat-sensitive (can not be sterilized by heat), you should replace it with a heat-tolerant or disposable alternative. If no heat-tolerant or disposable alternatives are available, use sterilant/high-level disinfectant to sterilize the item.
- **Noncritical patient-care items** for patient care include instruments and equipment that only contact intact skin. They have the lowest risk of disease transmission. Clean these items, or if visibly soiled, clean then disinfection with an EPA-registered hospital disinfectant. Alternatively, consider protecting these surfaces with disposable barriers.

Its risk of transmitting disease determines how a patient-care item is processed.
- Because they pose the greatest risk of disease transmission, critical patient-care items must be heat-sterilized.
- While semicritical items have a lower risk of disease transmission, most items in this category are heat-tolerant. Such instruments and supplies also should be heat-sterilized. Semicritical instruments that cannot tolerate the high temperatures of heat sterilization should be processed according to the manufacturer's instructions. This may include liquid sterilization, high-level disinfection or a combination of barrier protection and intermediate-level disinfection. To provide the highest degree of patient safety, consider replacing heat sensitive items with heat tolerant or disposable versions.
- In most cases, noncritical patient care items can be cleaned and then low-level disinfected. Low-level disinfectants destroy some viruses, fungi, and bacteria. Noncritical items that are visibly contaminated with blood should be cleaned and disinfected with an intermediate-level disinfectant before use on the next patient. Intermediate-level disinfectants have broader antimicrobial activity; they also are tuberculocidal. See Ch. 8, Environmental Infection Control, for more info on these disinfectant categories.

Heat sterilization of patient-care items involves a series of procedures — removing contaminated instruments from the treatment area, cleaning, packaging and labeling, sterilization, and storage and distribution — as well as routine monitoring of the sterilizer and the sterilization process. For items that are high-level disinfected, the process includes removing contaminated instruments from the treatment area, cleaning, immersion in a sterilant/high-level chemical disinfectant, aseptic preparation of items for storage or distribution at chairside, and monitoring and replenishing the disinfectant chemicals.

Terms You Should Know

Bioburden

Contact time

Disinfection

  High-level

  Intermediate-level

  Low-level

Exposure incident

Heat sterilization

Patient-care item(s)

  Critical

  Semicritical

  Noncritical

Sterilant

Sterilization

Sterilant/high-level disinfectant

Surfactant

Tuberculocidal

For definitions, see "Glossary," beginning on p. 166

The Bottom Line

Instrument processing requires a series of steps to assure that contaminated patient-care items are safe for reuse. All procedures must be performed correctly every time to make sure that items are processed properly and in the safest way possible. When processing contaminated instruments, always wear puncture-resistant utility gloves to prevent injury, and wear face and eye protection to protect against splash and spatter of contaminated materials.

* Dental handpieces touch mucous membranes but do not penetrate bone or soft tissue, so they are semicritical instruments. Although there is no evidence that handpieces have transmitted disease, they can pull oral fluids into their internal compartments (called "retraction" or "suck back"). In theory, fluids or debris retracted from one patient could be expelled later while treating another. To ensure patient safety, always sterilize handpieces using heat (for example, using an autoclave). For more on handpiece processing, see Ch. 10, Dental Handpieces and Other Devices Attached to Air and Waterlines.

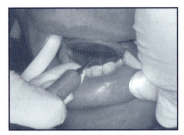

Instruments become contaminated with patient blood and oral fluids during treatment. Sterilize heat-tolerant items used intraorally.

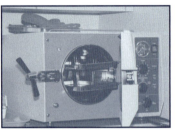

Most dental practices use autoclaves to process reusable patient-care items.

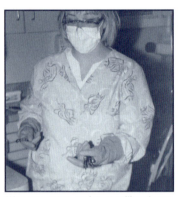

Wear puncture-resistant utility gloves when processing instruments.

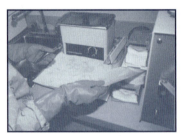

In the instrument processing area, keep supplies within easy reach.

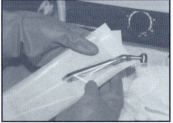

Package instruments before sterilization to protect them from contamination after the cycle.

Categories of Patient-Care Items

Category	Definition	Examples
Critical	Penetrate soft tissue, contact bone, enter into or contact the bloodstream or other normally sterile tissue	Surgical instruments, scalers, scalpel blades
Semicritical	Contact mucous membranes, but will not penetrate soft tissue, contact bone, or enter into or contact the bloodstream or other normally sterile tissue	Dental mouth mirror, amalgam condenser, reusable dental impression trays, dental handpieces, low speed motors, reusable prophy angles, digital radiography sensors, digital imaging wands
Noncritical	Contact with intact skin	Blood pressure cuff, stethoscope, pulse oximeter, face bow, radiographic head/cone

Digital X-Ray Sensors

Digital radiography sensors are semicritical items. Refer to manufacturer instructions for cleaning and reprocessing. Ideally, you should thoroughly clean these sensors and heat-sterilize or use a liquid sterilant between patients. If the sensor cannot tolerate these procedures, protect with an FDA-cleared barrier, clean the item, and disinfect with an EPA-registered hospital disinfectant with intermediate-level (i.e., tuberculocidal claim) activity, between patients.

All instruments, devices and other patient care items must be safe for patient use. Patient care items are either reusable, or single-use. Reusable items are instruments, devices or other items that can be appropriately cleaned, disinfected, or sterilized before use on another patient. Single-use items are not safe for use on more than one patient, often because the product design prevents, or the material cannot withstand cleaning, disinfection or sterilization.

Your practice should:

○ Have written policies and procedures to ensure that reusable instruments, devices or other items are cleaned and reprocessed appropriately before use on another patient.

○ Have manufacturer reprocessing instructions for reusable instruments and dental devices readily available, ideally in or near reprocessing areas.

○ Train DHCP responsible for reprocessing reusable dental instruments and devices at least annually and when new equipment or processes become available.

○ Provide training and equipment to ensure that DHCP wear appropriate PPE to prevent exposure to infectious agents or chemicals.

○ Label sterilized items with the sterilizer used, the cycle or load number, the date or sterilization and expiration date (if applicable).

○ Use only FDA-cleared medical devices for sterilization.

○ Perform routine maintenance for sterilization equipment according to manufacturer instructions and ensure maintenance records are available.

○ Have policies and procedures are in place to respond to reprocessing error or failure.

The Instrument Processing Area

Your practice should have a central instrument processing area divided into distinct "dirty" and "clean" areas. On the dirty side, you receive, clean, and decontaminate patient care items. Between the dirty and clean sides is the area used to prepare and package instruments for sterilization. On the clean side, instruments are sterilized and stored. If space doesn't allow for a separate instrument processing area, place "dirty" devices and supplies as far away from clinical contact surfaces as possible, and only process instruments when the area is not being used for patient care. Use signs to designate "dirty" and "clean" areas.

The instrument processing center should be set up so that as you walk patient-care items through receiving, holding, cleaning, preparing, packaging, sterilization, and storage, you move from the dirty side to the clean side. This contains contamination and helps make the process more efficient.

Work Flow Through the Instrument Processing Area

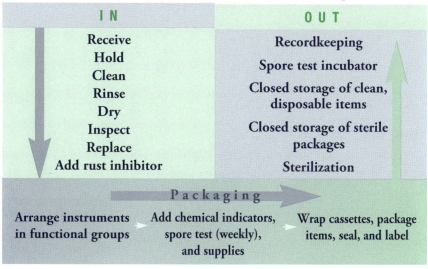

IN	OUT
Receive	Recordkeeping
Hold	Spore test incubator
Clean	Closed storage of clean, disposable items
Rinse	
Dry	Closed storage of sterile packages
Inspect	
Replace	Sterilization
Add rust inhibitor	

Packaging

Arrange instruments in functional groups	Add chemical indicators, spore test (weekly), and supplies	Wrap cassettes, package items, seal, and label

Move patient-care items from the "dirty" to the "clean" side of the instrument processing area.

Instrument Processing

Instrument processing requires a number of steps that must be performed correctly every time to make sure that items are properly processed. Your dental practice should have polices and procedures in place for instrument processing.

I.   Removing items from the operatory
To prepare the operatory for the next patient, contaminated materials must be safely removed and discarded or processed.

II.   Using holding solutions
If instruments can't be cleaned soon after use, place them in a holding solution.

III.   Cleaning
Cleaning is the most important step in instrument processing. To allow the sterilizing or disinfecting agent contact with all instrument surfaces, any remaining blood, body fluids, and other visible debris must be cleared away.

Two acceptable methods of instrument cleaning are manual (handscrubbing) and automated (ultrasonic cleaners and instrument washers). Automated methods are preferred over handscrubbing because they limit contact with contaminated instruments and in turn, the chance of an exposure.

Practice Tip

Hold It!

Hold instruments in solution to make them easier to clean later

If you can't clean them immediately, keep instruments moist to make sure they're still easy to clean when you're ready to do the job.

If debris is allowed to dry and harden on instrument surfaces, even automated cleaners can have a hard time removing it. And if instrument surfaces are not clean, your sterilizer may not be able to do its job.

Because the goal is only to keep debris moist, holding solutions don't need to have disinfectant properties.

Use an enzymatic presoak or cleaner. Enzymatic cleaners and presoaks are specially formulated to loosen debris.

Don't use a sterilant/ high-level disinfectant as a holding solution. Glutaraldehydes, for example, can bind debris to instrument surfaces, making cleaning even more difficult.

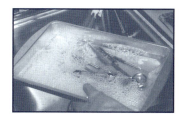

If instruments can't be cleaned soon after use, soak them to keep debris moist and easy to remove later.

Instrument Cassettes

Instrument cassettes are perforated stainless-steel, aluminum, or resin containers that hold instruments during all instrument processing procedures, from collection at chairside through sterilization and distribution for use on the next patient.

Instrument cassettes ...

○ ... **greatly reduce direct handling of contaminated instruments** and in turn, help prevent injuries.

○ ... **are available for all modes of heat sterilization**: autoclave, chemical vapor, and dry heat.

○ ... **minimize set-up time**. They contain instruments in functional sets from operatory teardown through cleaning, wrapping, sterilization, storage, and use on the next patient.

○ ... **hold instruments securely** so tips are not damaged during instrument processing.

○ ... **also can hold unit-dosed supplies** such as cotton gauze. Add them to the cassette after the cleaning, rinsing, and drying to eliminate the need to touch cabinets, drawers, and containers during treatment.

Ensure that cassettes are compatibly sized for your automated cleaner and heat sterilizer. Follow the manufacturer's instructions for cleaning, wrapping and bagging, and sterilization.

IV.   Preparing and Packaging

After cleaning, inspect instruments and other items; assemble them into sets or trays; and then wrap and package for heat sterilization. Remember that while the instruments have been cleaned of debris that could compromise the sterilization process, they are still contaminated with microorganisms, so keep your utility gloves on.

V.   Sterilization

In dental settings, heat-tolerant instruments generally are sterilized by steam under pressure (autoclave), dry heat, or unsaturated chemical vapor. Use only FDA-cleared devices that are designed for sterilization, and always follow the manufacturer's instructions for proper use.

VI.   Storing Sterile and Clean Patient-Care Items

Your practice setting has a choice as to how it maintains its instrument storage area. Event-related instrument storage and distribution recognizes that the contents of a sterilized package should remain sterile indefinitely unless some event — for example, torn or wet packaging material — causes it to become contaminated. Some facilities, however, store and use instruments on a "first in, first out" basis.

If available, use closed or covered cabinets to store dental supplies and instruments to keep sterile packs away from contaminants. Never store dental supplies and instruments under sinks or in other locations where they can become wet.

Cleaning Methods

Automated cleaning methods are preferred over handscrubbing. Automated cleaning — such as using an instrument washer or an ultrasonic cleaner — reduces your contact with contaminated instruments and in turn, the chance of an injury.

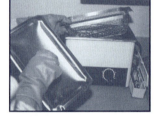

Ultrasonic cleaners use a special solution and high-energy sound waves to loosen and break up debris on instruments. The automated cycle reduces worker contact with contaminated items and frees staff to perform other tasks while the instruments are being cleaned efficiently and effectively.

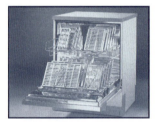

Instrument washers use high water flow rates and special detergents to safely and efficiently clean instruments. Fully automated, these units eliminate the need for pre-soaking, handscrubbing, rinsing, and drying and minimize contact with contaminated sharps. Some instrument washers also incorporate a high-level thermal disinfection cycle.

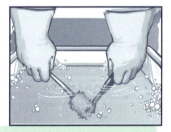

Handscrubbing puts workers in close contact with contaminated sharps and contaminated splash and spatter generated during the cleaning process. Handscrub instruments only when an automated cleaning process fails to remove stubborn debris.

Automated methods are preferred over handscrubbing. They reduce your contact with contaminated instruments and in turn, the chance of an injury.

Step by Step

Foil Testing Your Ultrasonic

Periodic testing is important for maintaining the cleaning effectiveness of your ultrasonic. Follow the manufacturer's recommendations for use of a commercially available soil removal test or follow the steps below for a simple foil test.

1 Use scissors to cut a piece of lightweight aluminum foil about the width of the ultrasonic cleaning tank and about an inch or so deeper.

2 Prepare a fresh tank of the cleaning solution you normally use in the ultrasonic unit. Fill to about 1-1/2 inches from the top of the tank.

3 Turn the unit on and set the timer to 5 minutes to degas.

4 When time has elapsed, insert the foil vertically into the tank. Hold the sheet of foil lengthwise across the long side of the tank and centered against the tank width. Extend the foil down toward the tank bottom. Do not let the foil touch the bottom of the tank.

5 Turn on the unit and hold the foil steady for exactly 20 seconds. When time has elapsed, turn off the cleaner, remove the foil, and carefully dry it, avoiding wrinkling.

6 Examine the foil sample. Uniform pitting and indentations across the part of the foil that was immersed indicates that the unit is delivering uniform cleaning power; smooth areas are a sign of ultrasonic "blind spots."

○ If you see uniform pebbling of the foil that was immersed, your unit is working properly.

○ In the case of blind spots, immediately retest the unit. If a second test confirms the presence of blind spots, schedule service. Sending the foil sample along with the repair request can help the technician locate the trouble spot.

Regular foil testing of your ultrasonic cleaner helps identify any mechanical problems that may arise. Consult the manufacturer for function tests specific to your unit.

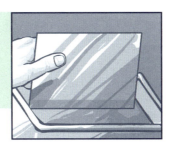

Step by Step

Wrapping Cassettes

After cleaning and prior to heat sterilization, wrap instrument cassettes in sterilization packaging material (see next page) and secure with heat-sensitive tape. Use a similar technique with instruments placed on a small sterilizable tray.

1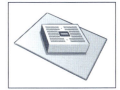

2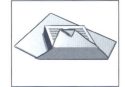

3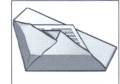

4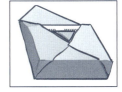

5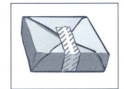

Sterilizing Agents for Heat Processes

Different methods of heat sterilization require different packaging materials because each uses a different sterilizing agent. A "sterilizing agent" creates the conditions in which microorganisms cannot survive.

❍ In an autoclave, pressurized steam is the sterilizing agent.

❍ As its name suggests, a chemical vapor sterilizer produces hot vapors of alcohol/formaldehyde as its sterilizing agent.

❍ In dry heat sterilizers, very high temperatures act as the sterilizing agent.

With all of today's sterilizers, exposure time and temperature are critical. Too short a contact time with the sterilizing agent can leave some microorganisms alive and well on instrument surfaces. Too low a temperature also can allow some pathogens to survive. As such:

❍ Always follow the sterilizer manufacturer's instructions for warming up and operating the unit.

❍ Never interrupt a sterilization cycle by opening the chamber door. If you must retrieve an item, start the cycle over from the beginning.

❍ To keep from contaminating them, allow instrument packs to dry inside the chamber before moving and handling them.

Packaging Patient-Care Items

To protect sterile instruments and supplies from contamination after the sterilization cycle, package cleaned instruments and fresh, nonsterile supplies before loading them into the sterilizer. Be sure to use only those packaging materials designed for use in your type of sterilizer. Improper packaging can melt, char, or even prevent the sterilizing agent from reaching the contents of the instrument packs.

Label each instrument pack with the date of sterilization, the sterilizer used, the cycle or load number, and the expiration date (if applicable). This will help retrieve processed items if a sterilization failure occurs. Never label packages with water soluble ink.

Packaging for Heat Sterilizing Patient-Care Items

	Packaging Material	Precautions
Steam autoclave	Paper wrap Nylon "plastic" tubing Paper/plastic peel pouches Thin cloth Wrapped perforated cassettes	No closed containers Thick cloth may absorb too much steam Some plastic containers melt Use only material approved for steam
Dry heat sterilizer	Paper wrap Appropriate nylon "plastic" tubing Closed containers Wrapped perforated cassettes	Some plastic containers melt Use only materials approved for dry heat
Unsaturated chemical vapor sterilizer	Paper wrap Paper/plastic peel pouches Wrapped perforated cassettes	No closed containers Cloth absorbs too much chemical vapor Some plastic containers melt Use only materials approved for chemical vapor

For autoclave or chemical-vapor sterilization, instruments may be placed in see-through paper/plastic pouches that are easily opened after sterilization.

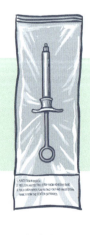

Heat Sterilization

In dental settings, heat-tolerant dental instruments generally are sterilized by steam under pressure (autoclave), dry heat, or unsaturated chemical vapor. Heat sterilizers are classified as medical devices and regulated by the U.S. Food and Drug Administration (FDA). This means that manufacturers of sterilizers must ensure that their devices meet performance criteria for safety and effectiveness.

Use devices that are intended only for heat sterilization and are cleared by the FDA. Review the manufacturer's instructions for use for recommended sterilization times, temperatures and other parameters. Also check the manufacturer's instructions for correct use of sterilization containers, wraps, pouches or other packaging that will be used with the sterilizer.

Use mechanical, chemical and biological monitors (discussed later in this chapter) and perform routine maintenance to ensure that your sterilizer is functioning properly.

> **Dental instruments and other patient care items should come with instructions for reprocessing.**
>
> **If the manufacturer does not provide instructions, then the item may not be suitable for use with multiple patients.**

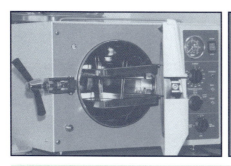
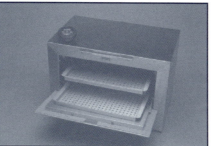

> **Autoclaves (left) and dry heat sterilizers (right) are commonly used to sterilize instruments and other patient-care items in dental settings.**

Flash Sterilization vs. Immediate-Use Steam Sterilization

"Flash" sterilization is an outdated term for a method used when urgently needed instruments were placed unwrapped into a steam sterilizer, allowing rapid contact with the steam. Today, the correct term is **Immediate-Use Steam Sterilization**. Immediate-use means the item is steam sterilized for a specific patient and procedure and used promptly upon removal from the sterilizer.

Immediate-use steam sterilization should only be used when there is an urgent need to sterilize an instrument that will be used immediately.

Never use immediate-use sterilization for implantable devices.

Immediate-use sterilization should not be used to save time or money spent on wrapping, or as an alternative to purchasing multiple sets of instruments.

If immediate-use steam sterilization is needed:

- Follow the sterilizer manufacturer instructions.
- Thoroughly clean and dry the instrument.
- Log all parameters (mechanical, chemical, biological) for each cycle.
- Handle hot, sterilized instruments carefully to avoid burns.
- Immediately and aseptically transport immediate-use sterilized items to the point of use.

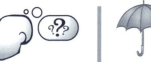

What If...

... a sterile instrument pack falls on the floor? Is it still sterile?

If you drop a sterile instrument pack, inspect the package for damage to the wrap or the contents. If packaging is compromised in any way — that is, if it is torn, punctured, or wet — repackage the contents in new packaging material and sterilize it again.

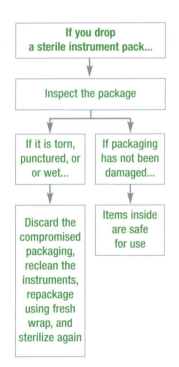

Storing Sterile and Clean Patient-Care Items

If available, use closed or covered cabinets to store dental supplies and instruments to keep sterile packs away from contaminants. Never store dental supplies and instruments under sinks or in other locations where they can become wet.

Use either date- or event-related storage. Date-related storage uses shelf life and the "first in, first out" principle to store and distribute sterile instrument packs. The event-related approach recognizes that the contents of a sterile package should remain sterile indefinitely, unless some circumstance — such as moisture or a tear in the packaging material — causes it to become contaminated.

Always inspect packages containing sterile supplies before use. If the package is moist, torn, or otherwise compromised, clean contents again, repackage using new wrap, and sterilize the items again.

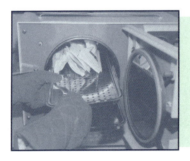

Wait for instrument packs to cool after the sterilization cycle. Handling hot and wet packages can transmit bacteria from the hands.

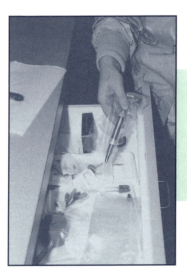

Sterile instrument packages that are cool and dry can be handled with clean hands.

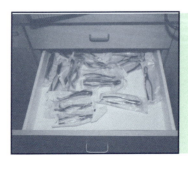

Store sterile instrument packages and clean patient-care items in closed or covered drawers or cabinets to protect them from droplet spatter and other contaminants.

Step by Step

Instrument Processing: Putting It All Together

All that you've learned so far about cleaning, preparing, packaging, steriliz-ing, and storage comes together to create a protocol for processing reusable patient care items.

Remove contaminated items from the operatory.

1 To prepare the operatory for the next patient, safely remove contami-nated materials. Discard all contaminated single-use disposable items (see "Managing Medical Waste," p. 70-72, for details on disposal).

2 Place reusable patient-care items in a leak-proof, puncture-resistant container with solid sides and bottom.

3 Cover the container to prevent accidental exposures.

4 Walk the container of contaminated reusable instruments to the desig-nated instrument processing area.

5 If instruments will be cleaned immediately, proceed to Step 9.

If instruments cannot be cleaned immediately, use a holding solution.

6 Once in the processing area, add a non-corrosive solution containing a surfactant — like an enzymatic presoak/cleaner — to the transport container.

— or —

Alternatively, don puncture-resistant utility gloves and carefully transfer the contaminated instruments from the transport container to a previous-ly prepared holding solution contained in a hard-walled, spill-proof con-tainer. Be sure the instruments are immersed in the solution.

❍ Change holding solution at least twice each day, more often if it is cloudy or visibly contaminated.

❍ Thoroughly clean and decontaminate the container on a routine basis.

When instruments are ready to be cleaned...

7 Don puncture-resistant utility gloves, face and eye protection, and protective apparel.

8 If you used a holding solution...

❍ Use forceps to remove loose instruments. Even with utility gloves in place, do not reach into the container with your hands.

❍ Rinse items under running water to remove solution and any loose debris from instrument surfaces. **NOTE**: Rinsing is important. Your holding solution may not be compatible with your automated cleaning unit.

Clean the instruments...

9 Proceed according to instructions for the method of cleaning you will be using: ultrasonic cleaning, instrument washer/washer-disinfector, or handscrubbing (see p. 54).

continued on p. 55

PPE in Processing Patient-Care Items

When processing contam-inated instruments, have puncture-resistant utility gloves, face and eye pro-tection, and protective ap-parel in place to prevent sharps injuries and splashes to skin, nose and mouth, eyes, and street clothes.

Thoroughly wash and dry hands after removing utili-ty gloves.

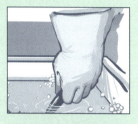
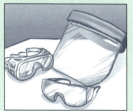
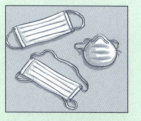
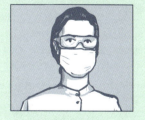
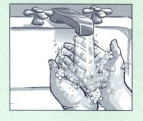

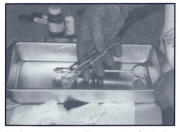

In the operatory, place contaminated reusable instruments in a leakproof, puncture-resistant container for transport to the processing area.

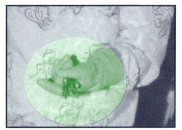

Always wear heavy-duty, puncture-resistant gloves when handling contaminated instruments.

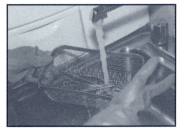

Rinse away holding solution before transferring instruments to an automated cleaning device.

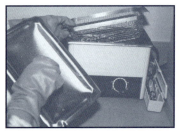

Use automated instrument cleaning methods, such as ultrasonic cleaners (above) or instrument washers.

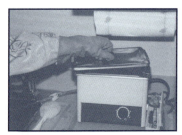

Always run the ultrasonic cleaner with the lid in place to reduce contaminated aerosols and droplets.

Cleaning Reusable Patient-Care Items and Instruments

Ultrasonic cleaner	Instrument Washer	Handscrubbing
○Follow the manufacturer's instructions for type and volume of solution to use, operation, cycle times, and maintenance.	○An instrument washer is not the same as a dish washer.	○Use a long-handled brush and a detergent that is not corrosive.
○Load the tank, being careful not to overload. Overloading can compromise cleaning performance and damage the unit.	○Follow the intructions provided by the manufacturer of your instrument washer.	○Place instruments low in the sink under running water. To ensure that you have the best control, clean no more than one or two instruments at a time, holding the instruments away from the sharp ends.
○Place the lid on the unit for the duration of the cycle.	○Proceed with processing (see next page). **NOTE**: Utility gloves must still be in place to reduce the risk of injury. Clean instruments are still considered contaminated with potentially infectious microorganisms.	○Inspect instruments for remaining debris. If necessary, scrub again.
○Rinse instruments or cassettes after the cycle.		○Allow instruments to air dry.
○Inspect instruments for remaining debris. If necessary, handscrub to remove.		**NOTE**: Utility gloves must still be in place to reduce the risk of injury. Clean instruments are still considered contaminated with potentially infectious microorganisms. *Never* rub instruments dry.
○Allow instruments to air dry, or carefully pat them dry with several thicknesses of towels. **NOTE**: Utility gloves must still be in place to reduce the risk of injury. Clean instruments are still considered contaminated with potentially infectious microorganisms. *Never* rub instruments dry.		○Proceed with reprocessing by packaging instruments for sterilization, sterilizing instruments, and storing/distributing them at chairside (see next page).
○Proceed with processing by packaging instruments for sterilization, sterilizing instruments, and storing/distributing them at chairside (see next page).		

Step by Step

Instrument Processing: Putting It All Together

continued from p. 53

Prepare and package instruments for heat sterilization

10 With utility gloves still in place, apply anti-corrosive agents as directed by the manufacturer of the instruments to be sterilized (for example, to non-stainless items that will be steam-sterilized).

11 Separate instruments into functional sets and add any patient care items that will be needed for treatment (such as cotton rolls or gauze).

12 Wrap, bag, or otherwise package instrument sets. Only use material that has been designed for use in heat sterilizers, and be sure the packaging material is compatible with the method of heat sterilization you will be using (autoclave, dry heat, or unsaturated chemical vapor).

13 Include a chemical indicator inside each instrument pack. Once per week, place a biological indicator (spore test) inside one instrument pack to be sterilized. (See "Sterilization Monitoring," p. 56-8.)

14 Seal each instrument pack. If the chemical indicator inside the package is no longer visible, place another on the outside of the pack. (See "Routine Sterilization Monitoring," p. 56.) Label the package as described on p. 50. Don't use water-soluble ink.

Sterilize the wrapped instruments

15 Load the sterilizer according to the manufacturer's instructions. Only use devices that are cleared by the FDA for sterilization. Do not overload the chamber.

16 Select and run the sterilization cycle. Check gauges for proper operating parameters (e.g., time, temperature, pressure). Do not open the chamber door while the sterilizer is operating.

17 After the cycle, allow instrument packets to dry (if sterilized using steam) and/or cool before handling.

18 Check chemical indicators for proper reaction. Retrieve biological indicators for incubation and analysis.

○ Do not use instrument packs if mechanical or chemical indicators suggest sterilizer malfunction.

○ If a spore test (biological indicator) comes back positive, follow instructions for "Troubleshooting a Sterilization Failure," p. 58.

Distribute or store sterile packs

19 Store sterile packs or distribute to chairside. Leave packaging intact until instruments are ready to be used in patient care.

20 Prior to use in patient treatment, inspect all packages containing sterile supplies to verify that the packaging material has not become torn, punctured, or wet. Damp packages are not considered sterile.

○ If a sterilized instrument pack is dry and intact, open it at chairside and use its contents during patient care.

○ If a sterile pack has been compromised, do not use the instruments inside for patient care. Instead, clean and repackage the instruments and subject the pack to another sterilization cycle.

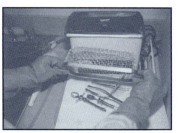

After the cleaning cycle, inspect items for residual debris and damage.

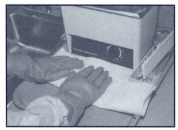

Wearing heavy-duty utility gloves, pat cleaned instruments dry under several layers of disposable paper towels.

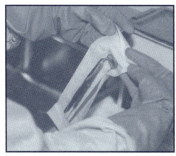

Pack and seal cleaned instruments in material that is compatible with the heat sterilizer. This pouch will be placed in an autoclave.

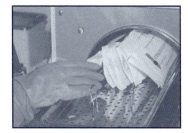

Load instrument packs in the sterilizer chamber. Leave room between packs so the sterilizing agent can contact all sides of every pack.

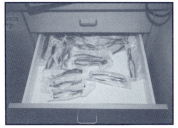

Store sterile instrument packs away from contaminants, preferably in a closed or covered cabinet or drawer.

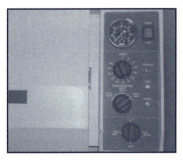
Check gauges during sterilization cycles.

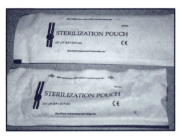
A color-change chemical indicator on the outside of the sterilization pouch identifies processed packs.

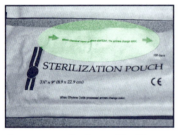
Arrows or a color change identify packets that have been heat sterilized.

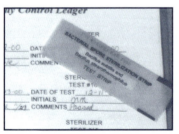
Supplied in strips (shown) or vials, biological indicators contain large numbers of highly resistant bacterial endospores.

Record results of sterilizer spore testing in the facility's sterilization monitoring log.

Sterilization Monitoring

Monitoring of sterilization procedures uses a combination of products and techniques that evaluate sterilizing conditions to ensure effectiveness of the procedure. Always consult manufacturers instructions for proper sterilization monitoring.

○ **Mechanical techniques** include assessing cycle time and temperature by observing gauges and displays during each load and examining the sterilizer's temperature record chart and computer printout, if available.

○ **Chemical indicators** monitor sterilization parameters such as time, temperature, and for autoclaves, pressure.

○ **Biological indicators** (BIs, or "spore tests") test the sterilization cycle by using heat-resistant organisms called bacterial endospores. If exposure to the sterilization cycle killed the spores, then less resistant microorganisms in numbers commonly found on dental instruments likely could not survive the process.

Routine Sterilization Monitoring

	Mechanical	Chemical	Biological
WHEN	With each load	With every instrument pack	At least weekly. All loads containing an implantable device
WHY	To detect gross sterilizer malfunction or improper loading	To identify sterilized from unsterilized instrument packs. To help detect gross sterilizer malfunction	To directly measure the sterilization process
HOW	Monitor cycle time and temperature: Examine temperature record charts and computer printouts, visually observe gauges, and assess pressure via the pressure gauge. Dynamic air removal sterilizers also may require an air removal test. Check with the manufacturer of your unit.	Place a chemical indicator on the inside of each package. If it is not visible from the outside, place an additional chemical indicator on the outside of the pack.	1. Subject a test biological indicator (spore test) to a normal sterilization cycle. 2. Incubate the test strip/vial alongside a control spore strip/vial from the same lot that has not been heat sterilized. 3. If the test strip/vial yields no growth and the accompanying control shows positive growth, it implies that the sterilization process killed the spores on the test strip.

Biological Monitoring

Biological monitoring is your best assurance that sterilization equipment is functioning and instrument processing procedures are being performed correctly.

Spore test weekly and when any changes are made to your sterilization procedures. For example:

❍ When a new packaging material is used

❍ After training new personnel

❍ Before initial use of sterilizers that have been:
  • Newly installed
  • Moved
  • Repaired

The type of spore used in sterilizer monitoring depends on the type of Sterilizer: *Geobacillus stearothermophilus* for autoclaves and chemical vapor units and *Bacillus atrophaeus* for dry heat.

Spore tests may be incubated using in-office incubation systems or by a mail-back monitoring service, such as those offered by some medical companies, universities, and dental schools. Although postal service delays can cause spore tests to arrive at the service many days after the sterilization process, mail delays do not influence spore incubation, growth, or final test results.

❍ For quality assurance, spore test your sterilizer(s) at least weekly.

❍ Use a test and a control strip/vial from the same manufacturer and lot.

❍ To reduce the risk of serious post-surgical infection, spore test with every load that contains an implantable device*. Whenever possible, do not surgically place the device until after the results of the biologic spore test are known.

❍ Use the correct spores for your sterilizer.

❍ If you analyze spore test results in-office, use the proper incubation temperature for the time specified by the manufacturer.

Always consult manufacturers instructions for proper sterilization monitoring.

* Most implantable devices are pre-sterilized by the manufacturer.

The Sterilization Monitoring Log

Record results of biological monitoring and keep sterilization monitoring records (mechanical, chemical, and biological) long enough to comply with regulations in your state or locality.

Your sterilizer log should include:

❍ Sterilizer identification number

❍ Sterilization date/cycle load

❍ Duration and temperature of sterilization cycle (if it is not recorded mechanically on a disk or chart)

❍ A description of the general contents of the load

❍ Operator's name

❍ Biological monitoring results for both test and control spores

❍ Repair and preventive maintenance (date, type of service)

❍ Blank area for notes (for example, different operator, load contents other than normal)

Biological Monitoring for Common Heat Sterilizers in Dentistry

	Spore	Incubation Temperature
Autoclave	*Geobacillus stearothermophilus*	56°C
Dry heat sterilizer	*Bacillus atrophaeus*	37°C
Chemical vapor sterilizer	*Geobacillus stearothermophilus*	56°C

What If ... ?

... a spore test indicates a sterilization failure? What should we do?

If the mechanical (time, temperature, pressure) and chemical (internal or external) indicators suggest a properly functioning sterilizer, a single positive spore test may not indicate sterilizer malfunction.

Most sterilization failures are due to human error, rather than to an equipment malfunction. Common causes of sterilization failure include overloading, inadequate space between instrument packs in the chamber, and use of improper or excessive packaging.

Use this flowchart and the chart on the next page to help you troubleshoot any sterilization failures encountered in your facility.

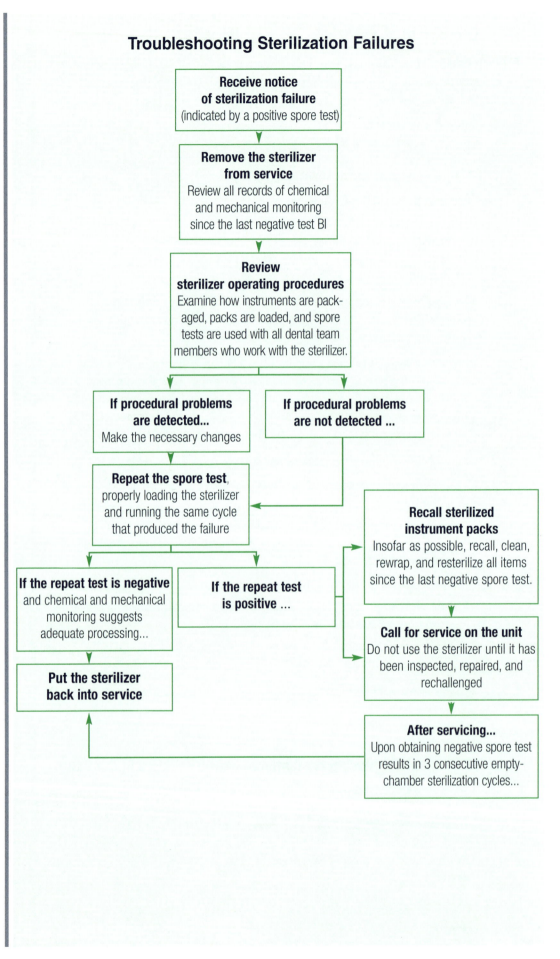

Common Causes of Heat-Sterilization Failure

Improper packaging

Wrong packaging material	Prevents penetration of sterilizing agent; packaging material may melt
Excessive packaging material	Retards penetration of the sterilizing agent
Cloth wrap in a chemical vapor sterilizer	Can absorb chemicals, preventing sufficient vaporization for sterilization
Closed container in steam or chemical vapor sterilizers	Prevents direct contact with the sterilizing agent

Improper loading of the sterilizer

Overloading	Increases heat-up time and retards penetration of the sterilizing agent to the center of the sterilizer load
Packages or cassettes loaded too close together, even without overloading	May prevent or delay contact of sterilizing agent with all items in the chamber

Improper timing

Incorrect operation of the sterilizer	Not enough time at proper temperature to achieve microbial kill
Timing for sterilization begun before proper temperature is reached (units with manual timers)	Not enough time at proper temperature to achieve microbial kill
Dry-heat sterilizer door opened during sterilizing cycle	Not enough time at proper temperature to achieve microbial kill
Sterilizer timer malfunction	Timer does not accurately reflect chamber conditions, resulting in insufficient time at proper temperature to achieve microbial kill

Improper temperature

Incorrect operation of the sterilizer	Not enough heat for proper time interval to achieve microbial kill
Sterilizer malfunction	Gauges do not accurately reflect chamber conditions, resulting in insufficient heat for proper time interval to achieve microbial kill

Improper method of sterilization

Solutions or water processed in a chemical-vapor sterilizer	Sterilizing agent does not penetrate the solution
Solutions or water processed in a dry heat sterilizer	Liquids boil over and evaporate
Processing heat-sensitive items	Items melt or distort

Sterilization Monitoring Summarized

◯ Use mechanical, chemical, and biological monitors to ensure the effectiveness of the sterilization process.

◯ Monitor each load with mechanical and chemical indicators.

◯ Place a chemical indicator on the inside of each package. If it is not visible from the outside, place another on the outside of the package.

◯ Do not use instruments if mechanical or chemical indicators suggest inadequate processing.

◯ Monitor sterilizers with biological test and control indicators at least weekly.

◯ Use a biological and control indicator for every sterilizer load that contains an implantable device. Verify results before using the device.

◯ In the case of a positive spore test, review sterilization procedures and follow the protocol outlined on p. 58.

◯ Maintain sterilization records (mechanical, chemical, biological) in compliance with state and local regulations.

Once instruments are bagged and ready, which way do the pouches go into the sterilizer?

First, review the manufacturer's instructions for your sterilization supplies and equipment. Generally, instrument pouches should be placed on edge in the sterilizer, facing the same direction (plastic facing paper).

Do not stack the pouches in a pile and do not overload the sterilizer.

Leave some room between each pouch to allow the sterilizing agent to contact all sides of each pouch.

Glass Bead / Salt Sterilizers

These small devices heated glass beads or salt to very high temperatures. When dipped into the beads, instrument tips, endodontic files and broaches were "sterilized."

However, there is no way to monitor these units or ensure the sterility of instruments. The FDA determined that these devices are neither safe nor effective and the devices are no longer marketed in the US.

Common Questions and Answers

All that information on heat sterilization is great, but how do we process patient-care items that are heat-sensitive?

With advances in instrument and equipment material and technology, very few items used in routine dental treatment today cannot withstand heat sterilization. Replacing heat-sensitive items with heat-tolerant or single-use disposable versions is the better infection control and safety choice.

The use of heat-sensitive patient care items and liquid chemical sterilants is discouraged for a number of reasons:

○ Some chemical germicide fumes irritate the skin, the mucous membranes of the eyes, and respiratory tissues. Several cases of occupational asthma among dental and other healthcare workers have been linked to glutaraldehydes.

○ Chemical sterilization cannot be verified with biological indicators.

○ Items that have been cleaned and then chemically sterilized must be rinsed with sterile water to maintain sterility and to remove toxic or irritating residues. Afterwards, the objects must be handled and dried with sterile gloves and towels and brought to chairside in a manner that maintains sterility. Items that have been chemically processed cannot be stored.

○ Use personal protective equipment when working with chemical sterilants, including chemically resistant gloves and aprons, goggles, and face shields. Although glutaraldehyde-based sterilants can be used safely, adverse effects have been reported. Skin sensitization also has been noted in some individuals.

○ Sterilizing instruments using liquid chemical germicides may require up to 12 hours of complete immersion; shorter soaking times are used to achieve high-level disinfection.

○ If liquid chemical sterilants must be used, manufacturer instructions must be followed closely. Follow manufacturer instructions regarding room exhaust ventilation.

We use barriers (surface covers) on our intraoral cameras and digital x-ray sensors. Is that all we need to do?

Newer "high-tech" dental equipment like digital x-ray sensors, lasers, intraoral cameras, electronic periodontal probes, and occlusal analyzers can vary in their ability to be sterilized or high-level disinfected.

During patient care, barrier-protect semicritical items that cannot be processed by immersion or heat sterilization, then clean and disinfect them between patients by using an intermediate-level disinfectant according to the manufacturer's instructions (see Ch. 8, Environmental Infection Control, for more info on intermediate-level disinfectants). Consult the device manufacturer on appropriate barrier and disinfection/sterilization procedures for the instrument or equipment in question.

Exercises in Understanding

1. Walk through your instrument processing area. Does the walk-through take you from a dirty to a clean side? If not, how could the area be rearranged to contain contamination?

   _____

   _____

2. Do you have all the proper personal protective equipment in place when handling and cleaning contaminated instruments?
   ❏ utility gloves   ❏ face and eye protection   ❏ protective apparel

3. What is your practice's protocol for storing wrapped instruments?

   _____

4. How are instruments typically cleaned in your practice setting?

   _____

5. How often does your practice spore test its sterilizers, and where are the results recorded?

   _____

Recommended Readings and Resources

CDC Health Alert Network. CDC/FDA Health Update about the Immediate Need for Healthcare Facilities to Review Procedures for Cleaning, Disinfecting, and Sterilizing Reusable Medical Devices. HAN 00383. OCT 2015. Available at: *emergency.cdc.gov/han/han00383.asp*

Centers for Disease Control and Prevention. Oral Health Resources: Frequently Asked Questions. Available at: *www.cdc.gov/OralHealth/infectioncontrol/faq/*.

Centers for Disease Control and Prevention. Guideline for Disinfection and Sterilization in Healthcare Facilities, 2008, Available at: *www.cdc.gov/hicpac/pdf/guidelines/Disinfection_Nov_2008.pdf*

Miller CH. *Infection Control and Management of Hazardous Materials for the Dental Team,* 6th edition St. Louis: Elsevier 2018.

Self-Test

Before moving on, test yourself with some questions on the material.
(answers appear below)

1. Placing contaminated instruments in a detergent solution or enzymatic cleaner to prevent debris from drying on their surfaces is called:
   a. holding   b. cleaning   c. sterilizing   d. storing

2. List three examples of a critical dental instrument.

   _____   _____   _____

3. List three examples of a semicritical dental instrument.

   _____   _____   _____

4. During instrument cleaning and packaging, wear _____ to protect your hands against sharps injuries.
   a. exam gloves   c. utility gloves
   b. sterile surgical gloves d. heat-resistant gloves

5. What type of indicators are placed inside each instrument pack of each cycle?
   a. biological   b. chemical   c. mechanical   d. all of the above

(1) a: (2) Surgical instruments, scalers, scalpel blades, surgical dental burs, endodontic files, any other instruments used to cut or penetrate bone or soft tissue: (3) Dental mouth mirror, amalgam condenser, reusable dental impression trays, dental handpieces, digital x-ray sensor, intraoral camera, dental laser, periodontal probe, explorer, any other instrument that contacts but does not penetrate mucous membranes: (4) c: (5) b.

Notes

Chapter 8

Environmental Infection Control

Examining the Issues

Environmental infection control addresses two main themes: managing contamination of surfaces, and proper handling and disposal of medical waste.

Surfaces in the dental operatory may become contaminated during patient care. Although contaminated surfaces have been linked to disease transmission in the hospital setting, environmental surfaces have never been associated with transmission of disease to patients, workers, or others within the dental setting.

Environmental surfaces — surfaces of equipment, furniture, walls, and flooring — are all considered noncritical surfaces. Environmental surfaces can be further categorized as either clinical contact surfaces or housekeeping surfaces.

○ **Clinical contact surfaces** are directly touched by contaminated instruments, devices, hands, or gloves. Use barriers to protect these surfaces from contamination during treatment, or clean and disinfect them between patients.

○ **Housekeeping surfaces** are not directly touched during the delivery of dental care. Unless they are visibly contaminated, they only require regular cleaning to remove soil and dust.

Environmental surfaces carry the lowest risk of disease transmission. As such, they can be managed using less rigorous methods than those used for dental patient-care items.

When using surface barriers to manage clinical contact surfaces, change barriers between patients. The surfaces under the barriers need only be cleaned and disinfected at the end of the clinic day unless they somehow become contaminated during treatment or removal. For clinical contact surfaces that are not covered during treatment, cleaning and low- to intermediate-level disinfection should be performed after each patient visit and at the end of the work day. Barriers must be used on surfaces that cannot be effectively cleaned.

Always consult equipment and device manufacturers for information on good choices for chemical germicides. Some laminates, upholstery, or other materials may not be compatible with all liquid chemical germicides.

Protect yourself against occupational exposure to infectious agents and hazardous chemicals.

○ Always wear personal protective equipment when performing environmental cleaning and disinfection procedures.

Medical waste (both regulated and unregulated) must be handled in a manner that poses no threat of disease transmission to the dental team, waste handlers, the environment, and the public at large.

The Bottom Line

Environmental surfaces have not been associated with disease transmission in the dental setting. Nevertheless, it is your responsibility as a dental care provider to reduce risk as much as possible. Use surface covers and proper surface disinfection techniques and materials to manage contamination and prevent the risk of cross-infection. Proper waste segregation, handling, and disposal reduces the risk of injury to you and your coworkers, waste handlers, and the public. Always wear task-appropriate personal protective equipment.

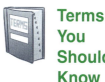

Terms You Should Know

Clinical contact surface

Disinfectant

Intermediate-level disinfectant

Low-level disinfectant

Environmental surface

Expiration date

Hepatitis B virus

HIV

Housekeeping surface

Medical waste

Noncritical

Personal protective equipment

Regulated medical waste

Sharps

Shelf life

Use life

For definitions, see "Glossary," beginning on page 166

Practice Tip

Use Surface Covers to Speed Operatory Turnaround

While infection control guidelines specifically suggest using surface barriers on hard-to-clean surfaces, there are big benefits to using covers on easy-to-clean surfaces, too.

Using covers on all clinical contact surfaces, including countertops and tray tables, can boost safety and efficiency. Changing barriers takes less time and requires no potentially irritating chemicals.

Surface barriers are available for use on almost any operatory surface. Impervious to moisture, plastic wrap, plastic sheets or tubing, and plastic-backed paper can be purchased precut and fitted for hoses, light handles, headrests, and more. Rolls of tear-off film can be used to protect larger surfaces.

Surface covers save the time and work required for cleaning and disinfection; they also eliminate the wait for the disinfectant contact times to elapse. Surfaces that remain covered during treatment need not be disinfected between patients. Just remove and replace the barrier.

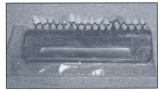

Covering the contact area of this shade guide eliminates the need to disinfect between patients.

Managing Clinical Contact Surfaces

Manage contamination of clinical contact surfaces either by covering them with surface barriers — highly recommended for difficult-to-clean surfaces — or by cleaning and disinfecting them between patients. Either method is effective. Most dental facilities seem to favor using a combination.

Barriers protect surfaces from becoming contaminated; between-patient cleaning and disinfection manages surfaces after they have become contaminated.

Step-by-Step: Using Surface Barriers

Apply an appropriate surface barrier to clinical contact surfaces before they have a chance to become contaminated.

! If surfaces to be covered are contaminated, clean and if necessary, disinfect them before placing new covers.

At the beginning of the clinic day, surfaces will have been cleaned at the end of the previous work day.

1 Apply an appropriate surface barrier to clinical contact surfaces before seating the first patient. Place each cover so that it protects the entire surface and will not be dislodged when touched.

Between patient visits...

2 Wear gloves when removing surface covers after patient treatment.
   ○ For simply removing contaminated barriers, the exam gloves worn during treatment are sufficient. Utility gloves also are acceptable.

3 Use care not to contaminate the surface underneath the barrier.
   ○ If the surface is touched when removing the cover (for example, with a contaminated glove or with the unclean side of the surface barrier), clean and disinfect the surface (see next page for instructions).
   ○ If the surface has not been touched with contaminated gloves or by the contaminated side of the cover, cleaning/disinfection is not necessary.

4 Discard used covers in the regular office trash unless your state or local disposal laws require special handling.

5 Remove and discard contaminated gloves, wash hands, and apply fresh surface covers (as directed in Step 1) for the next patient.

At the end of the clinic day....

6 Remove barriers and clean and disinfect all clinical contact surfaces in the operatory.

Categories of Environmental Surfaces

Category	Definition	Examples
Clinical Contact	Surfaces that are directly contacted by contaminated instruments, devices, hands, or gloves	Light handles, switches, dental x-ray equipment, reusable containers of dental materials, drawer handles, countertops, pencil, telephone handle, doorknob
Housekeeping	Surfaces that require regular cleaning to remove soil and dust	Floors, walls, sinks

Step-by-Step: Surface Disinfection

After each patient appointment, clean and disinfect all clinical contact surfaces in the operatory.

1 Put on utility gloves, mask, protective eyewear, and protective clothing to prevent contact with contaminants and chemicals through touching and splashing.

2 Determine the degree of cleaning/disinfection required and select a product compatible with the surfaces to be cleaned and disinfected.
   ○ For clinical contact surfaces not visibly contaminated with blood, select either a low-level disinfectant with HIV and HBV kill claims or an intermediate-level (tuberculocidal) disinfectant to clean and disinfect the surface. Follow germicide's label instructions for use.
   ○ For surfaces contaminated with blood or visibly bloody fluids, select an intermediate-level (tuberculocidal) disinfectant. Clean the surface then disinfect it according to the manufacturer's instructions.

3 Confirm that cleaning/disinfecting products have been prepared correctly and are fresh. Read and follow label instructions regarding dilution, shelf life, use life, and expiration date. Use only germicides that are registered with the Environmental Protection Agency (EPA) as hospital disinfectants.

4 Clean the surface.

   a Spray the surface with a cleaning agent.

   b Vigorously wipe with paper towels.
   ❏ When cleaning large areas, multiple surfaces, or large spills, use several towels to prevent transferring contamination from one surface to the next.
   ❏ Use a brush for surfaces that do not come visibly clean from wiping.

— or —

   a Wipe a premoistened cleaner-disinfectant towelette over the surface to be cleaned.
   ❏ Check the label to be sure that the wipe is a cleaner (some disinfectant wipes may require a separate cleaner).
   ❏ Carefully follow label instructions. Some wipes may be effective only on a limited surface area (approximately 3 sq. ft.).

5 After cleaning, disinfect the surface.

   a Spray the disinfectant over the entire surface, using towels to reduce overspray.

   b Let the surface remain moist for the contact time stated on the disinfectant's label.

   c Wipe the surface dry if it is still wet when ready for patient care.

— or —

   a Saturate the surface using a premoistened disinfectant towelette.

   b Let the surface remain moist for the contact time stated on the disinfectant's label.

   c Wipe the surface dry if it is still wet when ready for patient care.

Disinfecting Clinical Contact Surfaces

When using the "spray-wipe-spray" technique to clean and disinfect clinical contact surfaces use a low- (HBV/HIV kill) to intermediate-level (tuberculocidal) disinfectant.

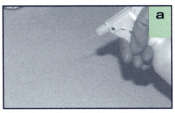

First clean, then disinfect. Spray the surface to be cleaned with a cleaner or cleaner/disinfectant...

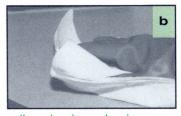

... then wipe vigorously using paper towels.

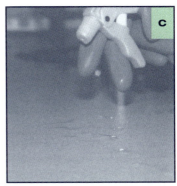

Once cleaned, spray the surface again, this time with a disinfectant. Cover the entire surface, and allow the disinfectant to remain undisturbed on the surface for the contact time indicated on its label.

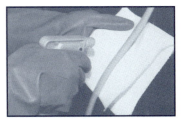

As needed, hold a paper towel in back of the surface to catch overspray, or adjust the pump spray nozzle to deliver a stream.

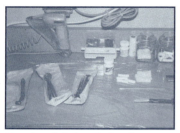

Covering clinical contact surfaces such as instrument trays and counter-tops prevents the surface beneath the barrier from contamination.

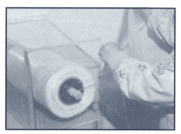

Surface barriers can be purchased in tear-off rolls for covering larger operatory surfaces.

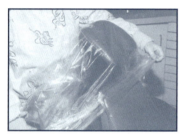

Covering the headrest before patient treatment eliminates the need to clean and disinfect it between patients.

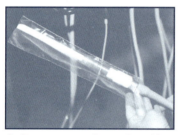

Surface covers can be purchased in "cut to fit" shapes and sizes to barrier-protect different instruments.

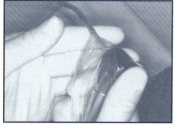

The handle of the air-water syringe is a clinical contact surface. Covering it protects it from contamination.

Covers vs. Cleaning and Disinfection

Using surface barriers is a safe, efficient way to protect operatory surfaces against contamination. Removing and replacing a surface barrier requires much less work and much less time than 'spray-wipe-spraying' clinical contact surfaces and waiting for the disinfectant contact time to elapse.

Cleaning and Disinfection *vs.* Using Surface Covers

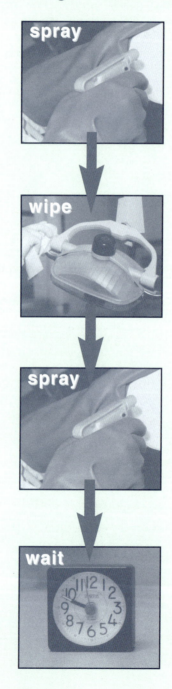

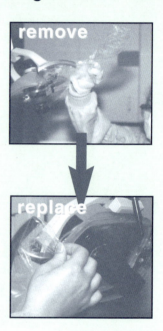

Managing Housekeeping Surfaces

There is no evidence that any bloodborne infection (HBV, HCV, or HIV) has been transmitted from a housekeeping surface (e.g., floors, walls) in a healthcare setting. Nonetheless, healthcare facilities should be kept clean.

Consult your practice setting's schedule for housekeeping procedures and follow it. Cleaning and disinfection schedules and methods may vary by area of the facility; that is, different housekeeping schedules may apply to the dental operatory, laboratory, bathrooms, and reception areas. Other factors that play a role in determining the housekeeping schedule include the type of surface and the amount and type of contamination it receives.

❍ On a regular basis and when visibly soiled, clean housekeeping surfaces with soap and water or an EPA-registered detergent/low-level disinfectant.

❍ When housekeeping surfaces are visibly contaminated, clean and decontaminate them using a low- or intermediate-level disinfectant immediately or as soon as feasible. However, after any spill of blood or other potentially infectious materials, use an intermediate-level disinfectant.

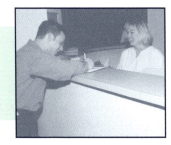

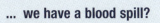
Establish a housekeeping schedule for treatment areas, lab, instrument processing, and reception areas.

What If ...

... we have a blood spill?

Most blood spills in dentistry are of a relatively small volume. Contain any blood spills on either clinical contact or housekeeping surfaces and manage them as quickly as possible to reduce the risk of contact and possible spread of contaminated materials to other areas of the practice setting.

1 Put on examination gloves and other personal protective equipment as needed.

2 Clean and decontaminate spills of blood or other potentially infectious materials using a low- to intermediate-level disinfectant, depending on size of spill and how porous the surface is.

a Check the germicide's label to ensure antimicrobial activity and surface compatibility.

b Remove visible organic material with disposable paper towels or other absorbent materials. Discard the towels in a leak-proof container color-coded red or labeled with the biohazard symbol.

c Clean and then decontaminate the non-porous surface with either a low-level disinfectant effective against HBV and HIV or an intermediate-level disinfectant.

Did You Know...?

... that carpeting is a warm and welcoming home to microorganisms?

It's true! Researchers have found diverse populations of microorganisms thriving in carpeting.

Carpeting also is harder to clean than hard-surface flooring, and there's no way to reliably disinfect it, especially after spills of blood and body substances.

Cloth furnishings pose similar contamination risks in areas of direct patient care and in places where contaminated materials are managed, like the dental operatory, lab, and instrument processing area.

As such, it's a good idea to avoid carpeting and fabric-upholstered furnishings in the dental setting. Smooth, nonporous, easy-to-clean flooring and upholstery is the better choice.

Clean and Disinfect

Follow the manufacturer's instructions for use for cleaning and disinfecting surfaces.

**In general:
When using spray—**

1. Spray disinfectant onto the surface

2. Wipe to clean visible or nonvisible debris

3. Allow surface to remain wet for the time indicated by the manufacturer for disinfection

When using premoistened disinfectant wipes—

1. Wipe surfaces to clean visible or nonvisible debris

2. Using fresh wipes, wipe surfaces to apply disinfectant

3. Allow surface to remain wet for the time indicated by the manufacturer.

Common Questions and Answers

What's the difference between a low-level and an intermediate-level disinfectant?

Unfortunately, your disinfectant labels won't say "low-level" or "intermediate-level" on them, so you're going to have to read between the lines a bit.

A low-level disinfectant will state on its label that it is a hospital disinfectant. This means that it is effective against the test microorganisms *Salmonella choleraesuis*, *Staphylococcus aureus*, and *Pseudomonas aeruginosa*. Any hospital disinfectant can be used on housekeeping surfaces that are not visibly contaminated with blood.

Some low-level hospital disinfectants also have a HBV and HIV kill claim. In addition to housekeeping surfaces, these products can be used to clean and disinfect clinical contact surfaces that are not visibly contaminated with blood.

An intermediate-level disinfectant is a hospital disinfectant that also is tuberculocidal (that is, it kills the hearty test microorganism *Mycobacterium tuberculosis*). Use intermediate-level disinfectants to disinfect clinical contact surfaces with or without visible blood. Intermediate-level disinfectants also are used to disinfect blood-contaminated housekeeping surfaces.

Always follow the disinfectant manufacturer's instructions for cleaning surfaces prior to disinfecting them.

How do we know which surface disinfectant is the best choice for our practice setting?

Because every practice setting is different, no one disinfectant is the best choice for every dental facility. Read disinfectant labels carefully and look for the following:

○ EPA registration number;

○ a "hospital disinfectant";

○ compatibility with surfaces, conditions of use, and staff who will use it;

○ cleaning as well as disinfecting properties (for easier inventory management);

○ low allergenicity;

○ ease of use;

○ clear, easy-to-follow instructions;

○ a reasonable contact time (i.e., less than 10 min.);

○ acceptable storage and disposal requirements; and

○ a reasonable use life and shelf life.

With regard to antimicrobial activity, consider the following:

Contamination	Clinical contact surfaces	Housekeeping surfaces
No blood	Hospital disinfectant plus (a) HBV and HIV kill claim or (b) tuberculocidal activity	Hospital disinfectant or detergent and water
Blood	Hospital disinfectant plus tuberculocial activity	Hospital disinfectant with tuberculocial activity

What else do we need to know about our surface disinfectants?

In addition to kill claims, the disinfectant label also identifies any hazards the chemical may pose (for example, it may be corrosive or toxic) and the precautions to take to protect yourself and your practice setting from those hazards.

On low- and intermediate-level disinfectant labels, you will find:

○ antimicrobial activity of the agent when used as directed (for example, a disinfectant may be virucidal, bactericidal, fungicidal; tuberculocidal; some may also list specific microorganisms);

○ active ingredients;

○ the necessary contact time for inactivation;

○ directions for use (including recommendations for cleaning surfaces before disinfecting);

○ precautionary statements;

○ storage and disposal instructions, shelf life, use life, and expiration date; and

○ EPA registration number (required for all hospital disinfectants sold in the United States).

Exercises in Understanding

1. With a coworker or your Infection Control Coordinator, walk through a typical patient exam, counting the number of surfaces that are contacted by contaminated gloves, instruments, and even droplet spatter.

2. Does your practice setting use between-patient surface disinfection, barriers, or a combination of both to manage contamination of environmental surfaces? Discuss the rationale of your practice setting's protocols with your Infection Control Coordinator.

   a) How long does it take to clean and/or disinfect an operatory? Be sure to include the time it takes to put on the appropriate protective equipment and the contact time required for the disinfecting agent to be effective.

   b) How long does it take to remove and replace barriers after patient treatment?

3. What is the housekeeping schedule in your practice setting for walls, floors, and other surfaces in:

   the dental operatories _____

   the reception area _____

   the instrument processing area _____

   the x-ray developing area _____

   the dental lab area _____

What's Regulated Medical Waste?

Examples of regulated waste in the dental setting include:

Sharps
○ Needles
○ Scalpel blades
○ Orthodontic bands and wires
○ Broken metal instruments
○ Burs

Blood and blood-saturated waste
○ Gauze
○ Cotton rolls

Pathological waste
○ Extracted teeth
○ Biopsy specimens
○ Surgically removed hard and soft tissue

Keep these waste products separate from the regular office trash. Your practice setting should have protocols in place to comply with state and local waste disposal requirements.

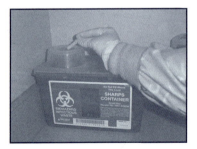

Keep contaminated sharps such as burs, needles, and scalpel blades separate from the rest of the facility's waste. Keep a sharps container in each operatory, and replace sharps containers as soon as contents reach the "fill" line on the container.

Managing Medical Waste

Although any item that has had contact with blood or secretions may be infectious, not all waste contaminated with blood or body fluids requires special disposal. Federal, state, and local guidelines and regulations specify which categories of medical waste are subject to regulation, and they outline any requirements for treatment and disposal.

Some examples of regulated waste found in a dental office are:
○ solid waste that is soaked or saturated with blood or body fluids (for example, gauze saturated with blood following surgery), or caked with dried blood;
○ extracted teeth, surgically removed hard and soft tissues; and
○ sharp items (for example, needles, scalpel blades, wires).

Managing Regulated Medical Waste: General Recommendations

○ Use a leak-resistant biohazard bag to contain "non-sharp" regulated medical waste.
  ❑ The bag must be color-coded red or identified by the biohazard symbol. Securely close the bag for disposal.
  ❑ Use care to ensure that discarded waste does not contaminate the bag's exterior.
○ Place sharp items in puncture-resistant biohazard containers. Close containers immediately before removing or replacing them to prevent contents from spilling or protruding during handling, storage, transport, or shipping.
  ❑ To reduce handling of contaminated sharps and in turn, the potential for injury, keep puncture-resistant sharps containers at the point of use — that is, in each operatory — to contain scalpel blades, needles, syringes, and unused sterile sharps.
  ❑ Do not recap, bend, break, or otherwise manipulate needles with unprotected hands. If recapping is necessary, use the one-handed scoop technique or an appropriate mechanical device to hold the needle cap away from your hands.
  ❑ When sharps containers are filled to the indicated capacity, close them securely and remove them from the operatory for final disposal. Never overfill a sharps container!
○ Do not dispose of extracted teeth containing amalgam in a container that will be incinerated. High temperatures release mercury vapor from amalgam, creating a hazard.
○ Your facility should dispose of medical waste regularly; it should not be allowed to accumulate within the practice setting.
○ Check with your Infection Control Coordinator for details on your facility's regulated medical waste management plan. The plan must comply with all federal, state, and local regulations.

What If ...

... the outside of the biohazard bag becomes contaminated?

If the outside of the biohazard bag used to contain nonsharp regulated waste becomes contaminated, simply place the contaminated bag inside a second biohazard bag. Do not reach in and transfer the contents.

Step by Step

Managing Regulated Medical Waste in the Dental Practice Setting

Managing regulated medical waste within the dental office should not be difficult; it's simply a matter of "divide and conquer."

1 **Handle**. To prevent exposure to contaminated materials, always use proper personal protective equipment when handling regulated waste.

❍ When handling solid sharps, wear utility gloves.

❍ When handling blood- or body-fluid-soaked or -caked materials, wear utility gloves, eye and face protection, and a protective garment.

❍ When handling extracted teeth, wear patient-care or utility gloves.

2 **Segregate.** Regulations for disposal are waste-specific, so separate waste when and where it is created to minimize handling and simplify disposal.

❍ Place any needles, burs, orthodontic bands and wires, and other disposable sharps in the sharps container.

❍ Red-bag any blood-saturated or -caked waste.

❍ Dispose of extracted teeth and tissues as required (see Ch. 17, Handling Extracted Teeth, p. 115-117).

3 **Store** securely sealed containers of regulated waste until they can be picked up by the contracted medical waste hauler or processed in the practice.

❍ Use rigid, leak-resistant containers that are impervious to moisture, strong enough to ensure they will not be damaged during handling, and sealed to prevent leaking.

4 **Label** containers clearly to guard against unintentional contact and exposure.

❍ The biohazard symbol identifies infectious waste. Your waste hauler will provide you with information on how to label toxic and other types of waste.

5 **Dispose** of regulated medical waste according to federal, state, and local requirements.

❍ Check with your state Environmental Protection Agency. Your state dental board may also have some helpful information.

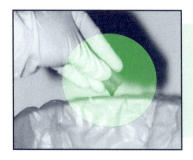

If an item releases blood under pressure, it is considered 'blood-soaked' and classified as regulated waste.

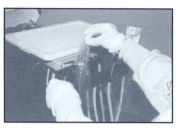

Although they may be contaminated with patient blood or body fluids, used surface covers are not regulated waste. Dispose of them in the regular office trash.

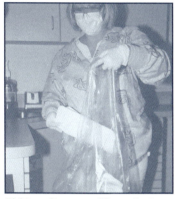

Divide and conquer: After patient treatment, collect items that can be discarded with the regular office trash. Place regulated waste...

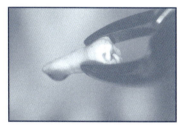

... like extracted teeth ...

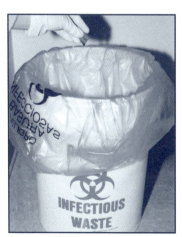

... and blood-soaked cotton or gauze, in an infectious waste container with a secure lid. Most facilities use a waste hauler to dispose of regulated waste.

Sharps Containers

According to the National Institute of Occupational Safety and Health (NIOSH), sharps containers should be:

❍ Closeable, puncture-proof, and leakproof on side and bottom.

❍ Easily accessible and located as close as is feasible to area being used.

❍ Labeled with the universal biohazard symbol and/or color-coded red.

❍ Designed so that users can see how full it is and when it needs to be replaced.

❍ Upright, not easily knocked over, and positioned so users have a clear, unobstructed view of the container opening.

❍ Located within arm's reach and placed at a height that is below eye level for users (typically 52-56 in. from the floor when wall-mounted, 38-42 in. for a seated workstation).

❍ Removed by staff and replaced when 3/4 full (as indicated by their "fill to" line).

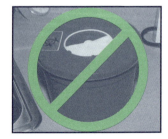

This sharps container has no fill line and contents are not visible.

Sterilizing Infectious Waste In-House

Some facilities use a medical waste hauling and disposal service, but these services can be very costly.

In areas where it is permitted by law, healthcare facilities can sterilize their filled sharps containers prior to disposal so that the contents are made nonhazardous. Check with your state medical waste agency to be sure this practice is allowed.

If your facility treats medical waste to make it safe for disposal, it should have a written procedure that contains clear, step-by-step instructions.

To sterilize filled sharps containers:

❍ Never heat sterilize sharps containers that hold extracted teeth containing amalgam. The high temperatures release mercury vapor from the amalgam, creating a hazard.

❍ Use an autoclave or chemical vapor sterilizer. Place the sharps container upright in the chamber (to prevent sharps from spilling out) with the vents open, and set the sterilizer to an extended exposure time of 40 to 60 minutes. Consult with the manufacturer of the sharps container for specific instructions.

❍ Following the cycle, allow the container to cool, then close the vents and label and dispose of the container as required by law.

❍ Monitor sterilizer efficacy with a biological indicator (spore test) for each load of waste processed. Add results of spore tests to the written record of waste processing.

❍ Maintain written records of waste processing, including the name of the operator, the method of sterilization, and the date. Also indicate the temperature and dwell time (the time chamber contents remained at the sterilizing temperature/pressure). Keep records for 3 years or as required by state and local regulations.

NOTE: Because of variations in waste management programs, consult your state agencies before implementing an in-office medical-waste treatment protocol. A special permit may be required.

Disposing of Blood and Other Body Fluids

Containers of blood or suctioned fluids may be sterilized in compliance with state-approved treatment technologies, or contents can be carefully poured down a utility sink drain or toilet if your local law permits.

There is no evidence that bloodborne diseases can be transmitted from contact with raw or treated sewage. Many bloodborne pathogens, particularly viruses, are not stable in the environment for long periods of time, so discharging small quantities of blood and other body fluids into the sanitary sewer is a safe and acceptable way of disposing of these waste materials.

State or local regulations may limit the maximum volume of blood or other body fluids that may be discharged into the sanitary sewer. Consult your infection control manager for details on regulations and limitations in your area.

Exercises in Understanding

1. Walk through your practice setting. Is a sharps container located in every operatory or lab where contaminated sharps are used?

2. Take a good look at the sharps containers used in your practice setting.

Are they color-coded red or labeled with the biohazard symbol?	❏ Yes	❏ No
Are contents of the container visible?	❏ Yes	❏ No
Do they have a clearly identifiable fill-to line on the outside?	❏ Yes	❏ No
Do they have lids that close and lock securely for transport?	❏ Yes	❏ No
Are they upright and securely mounted or seated to prevent spills?	❏ Yes	❏ No
Are they out of reach of children?	❏ Yes	❏ No

Self-Test

Before moving on, test yourself with some questions on the material.
(answers appear below)

1. If the outside of a biohazard bag becomes contaminated:
   a. heat sterilize it
   b. disinfect the surface of the bag
   c. throw it in the regular trash
   d. place it inside another biohazard bag

2. List three examples of a regulated waste in the dental setting.

   _____ _____ _____

3. The handle of the overhead operatory light is a _____ surface.
   a. housekeeping   b. clinical contact   c. porous   d. all of the above

4. What color indicates a biohazard?
   a. red   b. blue   c. yellow   d. green

5. An appropriate low-level disinfectant for dental settings will be effective against:
   a. *Mycobacterium tuberculosis*
   b. *Mycobacterium avium* complex
   c. HBV and HIV
   d. all of the above

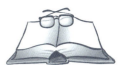

Recommended Readings and Resources

Centers for Disease Control and Prevention. Oral Health Resources: Frequently Asked Questions. Available at: *www.cdc.gov/OralHealth/infectioncontrol/faq/*

Healthcare Environmental Resource Center. Dental Offices – Regulated Medical Waste. Available at: *www.hercenter.org/dental/index.cfm*

National Institute for Occupational Safety and Health. *Selecting, Evaluating, and Using Sharps Disposal Containers*, DHHS (NIOSH) Pub. No. 97-111), January 1998. Available at: *www.cdc.gov/niosh/docs/97-111/*

Miller CH. *Infection Control and Management of Hazardous Materials for the Dental Team,* 6th edition St. Louis: Elsevier, 2018.

OSAP. Surface Disinfectant Reference Chart – 2014 Available at: *www.osap.org*

OSAP. Managing patient-care items and environmental surfaces. (Appendix C). *From Policy to Practice OSAP's Guide to the Guidelines.* Annapolis, Md.:OSAP, 2004:142.

OSAP. If Saliva Were Red: A Visual Lesson on Infection Control. *www.osap.org*

(1) d; (2) Any contaminated sharp, blood and blood-saturated or -caked waste materials, pathological waste, or hazardous waste including but not limited to needles, scalpel blades, orthodontic bands and wires, broken metal instruments, burs, blood-soaked or caked gauze or cotton rolls, extracted teeth, biopsy specimens, surgically removed hard and soft tissue, scrap amalgam, x-ray developer and fixer, chemical-vapor sterilizer solution, x-ray shields; (3) b; (4) a; (5) c.

Notes

Chapter 9

Dental Unit Waterlines, Biofilm, and Water Quality

Examining the Issues

In many dental settings, water used for dental treatment comes from the municipal water supply, through the office plumbing and directly into the dental unit. Thin, plastic tubing carries water from the dental unit to the highspeed handpiece, air-water syringe, ultrasonic scaler, and into the patient's mouth. The inside surface of these dental waterlines can become colonized with a variety of microorganisms, including bacteria, fungi, and protozoa that live inside a slime layer that protects and feeds them. This phenomenon, called a biofilm, allows microorganisms to survive and thrive in dental waterlines and raises concerns about possible health effects of exposure to bacteria and other organisms in dental unit water.

Biofilm forms in all water environments. The structure of narrow-bore dental tubing and the typical way dental unit water is used in the practice setting, however, worsens the problem.

○ Dental waterlines hold only a small volume of water, but the narrow diameter of the tubing results in a relatively large surface area for bacterial attachment and the formation of biofilm. Once formed, the biofilm serves as a reservoir that can increase the number of free-floating microorganisms in water used for dental treatment.

Microbial counts in dental treatment water can reach as high as 200,000 CFU/mL within 5 days of installing new dental unit waterlines. Counts greater than 1,000,000 CFU/mL have been reported.

Although oral flora and some human pathogens have been found living in dental water systems, most organisms recovered from dental waterlines are common water bacteria that have little potential for causing illness in healthy, immunocompetent persons. However, in recent years a number of cases of human illness and deaths associated with contaminated water from dental equipment however have been reported.

○ In two separate outbreaks, Georgia (2015) and California (2016) a total of nearly one hundred pediatric dental patients developed *Mycobacterium abscessus* post-treatment infections requiring hospitalization after exposure to contaminated water from dental units.

○ A fatal case of Legionella pneumonia in an elderly woman in Italy was reported in 2014. Investigators traced the origin of the Legionella species to water from dental units where the patient had received recent treatment.

○ In 2017, a second fatal case of Legionellosis was reported in Sweden. An elderly, immunocompromised patient treated in a hospital dental clinic became infected. Isolates from the dental unit cup-filler used for oral rinsing strongly suggested that they were of common origin.

Dental unit water that remains untreated is likely to contain high numbers of microorganisms and unlikely to meet drinking water standards. Use available commercial devices and procedures that improve the quality of dental treatment water to standards set by the Environmental Protection Agency (EPA) for safe drinking water under the surface water treatment rule (less than 500 CFU/mL).

The Bottom Line

Exposing patients or dental workers to water of poor microbiological quality is simply not consistent with accepted infection control principles. As such, dental practices should work with equipment manufacturers to ensure that their dental treatment water meets or exceeds the standards set by the EPA for drinking water.

Terms You Should Know

Biofilm

Colonize

Colony-forming units per milliliter (CFU/mL)

Filter

Flushing

Immunocompetent

Immunocompromised

Retraction

Self-contained water system

Waterline

For definitions, see "Glossary," beginning on p. 166

Commercially Available Water Quality Systems

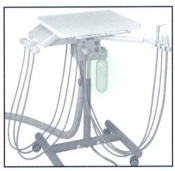

Self-contained water systems supply solutions from a reservoir (not the public water supply) filled and maintained by dental team members.

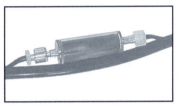

Some in-line filters combine filtration with continuous chemical release.

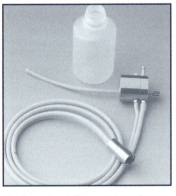

Sterile water delivery systems bypass the dental unit water supply completely. Their bottles, tubing, and connectors are autoclavable to ensure that sterile solutions are not contaminated before reaching the patient.

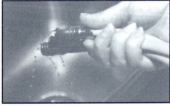

Flushing is not a reliable way of controlling dental water quality. Its effects are only temporary, as bacteria continually break off from the biofilm into treatment water.

Improving Dental Water Quality

Dental unit water that remains untreated or unfiltered is not likely to meet drinking water standards. To control and maintain the quality of dental unit water:

○ **Contact the manufacturer** of your dental unit to find out which method(s) of water quality control are compatible with your unit. Always follow the manufacturer's instructions for using any waterline maintenance product or protocol. Follow the schedule for maintenance and monitoring set forth by the manufacturer, except where it is inconsistent with local laws or regulations.

○ **Use commercial devices and procedures** designed to improve the quality of water used in dental treatment. Methods shown to be effective include:
  ❑ self-contained water systems that can be used with other available methods, including:
     ❑ Intermittent chemical treatment with germicidal agents or cleaners designed to inactivate and remove biofilm (shock treatment)
     ❑ Continuous treatment of water systems with low levels of a germicidal agent with active ingredients safe for human consumption and compatible with dental materials (iodine, silver) that are added to dental water reservoirs at chairside or introduced using pick up tubes with slow release germicide impregnated resin.
  ❑ in-line systems connected to municipal water that use slow release germicide impregnated resin or other technology to add metered amounts of germicide to water entering the dental unit.

Currently, removal or inactivation of biofilms in dental water lines requires the use of chemical germicides. Other technologies may become available in the future.

○ **Use source water containing less than 500 CFU/mL of bacteria** (for example, tap, distilled, or sterile water). In most urban areas, municipally plumbed water meets this standard. It is not uncommon however, for tap water quality to vary considerably over time and by location. Tap water quality can also be influenced by use of faucet aerators and issues with premise plumbing such as dead legs where bacterial biofilms can flourish. On-site distillers and reverse osmosis systems may provide water of acceptable quality, but the devices, tubing and reservoirs can also become contaminated over time and should be monitored and maintained. Bottled sterile water for irrigation provides the greatest margin of safety but cost consideration may make it impractical in most settings. Commercial bottled drinking water is a regulated product that is supposed to meet drinking water standards for bacterial contamination, but quality may be variable.

○ **Source water control alone will not eliminate contamination in treatment water if biofilm in the water system is not controlled.** Using source water of acceptable quality is critical, but will not ensure that water used in dental procedures is free from microbial contamination unless biofilm is controlled or eliminated from all components of the water delivery system including water reservoirs and external storage containers.

○ **Clean self-contained water systems** according to the manufacturer's instructions. Improperly maintained, these devices can become highly contaminated.

○ **After each patient, run any dental device used in the mouth and connected to the dental water system** for a minimum of 20-30 sec. to discharge water and air. Running handpieces, ultrasonic scalers, and air-water syringes after use physically flushes out any patient material that may have entered the turbine, air, or waterlines.

○ **Do not rely on flushing waterlines at the beginning of the clinic day to maintain water quality.** Flushing does not affect biofilm in the waterlines or reliably improve the quality of water used during dental treatment. Dental workers may wish to flush lines before beginning patient appointments for the day to clear stagnant water from the lines, but flushing is no longer recommended as a water quality-control measure.

◯ **If using a dental unit that is more than 30 yrs. old, consult the owner's manual or contact the manufacturer to determine whether anti-retraction valves or other devices are (or should be) present** and require testing or maintenance. Most recently manufactured dental units are engineered to prevent retraction of oral fluids, but older systems often have valves that require periodic maintenance. Even with anti-retraction valves, flushing the above devices for a minimum of 20-30 sec. after each patient is recommended.

Water Quality Controls: Pros and Cons

Type of Device	(+)	(-)
Self-contained water systems Isolate the dental unit from the municipal water supply, instead providing water or treatment solution from reservoirs filled and maintained by office staff.	Isolate the dental unit from the municipal water supply. Allow the practice to control the quality of water that is used in the unit. Provide a way to introduce chemical agents to waterlines and permit the use of water of known microbiologic quality.	Cannot reliably improve the quality of dental unit water without additional chemical or mechanical treatment against the biofilm within the unit. Improperly maintained, could deliver water of worse quality than from a municipal source (for example, if the reservoir becomes contaminated).
Chemical treatments Used with a self-contained reservoir, metering device, or water conditioning system. Depending on the specific product, used either periodically (in regular intermittent applications, or as a "shock" treatment) or as a continuous presence in the waterline.	Inactivate or prevent biofilm in dental waterlines.	When done manually, may be time-consuming and technique-sensitive. (Periodic disinfection involves purging the waterlines, adding a chemical to the water reservoir, filling the lines for the recommended time period, and flushing.) Requires strict compliance with the recommended treatment regimen. Products must be compatible with dental equipment. (The proper treatment protocol depends on the type and components of the dental unit.) Possible incompatibility between continuous-release chemicals and various dental materials (for example, dental adhesives).
Flushing Clears waterlines of free-floating microorganisms.	Between patients (for 20-30 seconds), helps to remove contaminants that may have been retracted during patient treatment.	Not a control method for dental water quality. Effects are only temporary (biofilm bacteria continually break free and recontaminate dental unit water during the course of clinical treatment). Alone, has little effect on waterline contamination. Does not prevent or eliminate biofilm.
Sterile Water Delivery Systems Self-contained water systems with disposable or autoclavable tubing that bypasses the dental unit's water supply.	Delivers sterile water to the patient when a sterile water source is used. Available for oral-surgery and implantology handpieces, ultrasonic scalers, and retrofit devices for restorative handpieces.	Autoclavable components require sterilization between uses.

Sterile Surgical Irrigation

To help guard against post-surgical infection:

❍ **Use only sterile water or sterile saline as a coolant/irrigant for surgical procedures** that involve incision, excision or reflection of tissue exposing previously sterile areas of the oral cavity.

❍ **Use only sterile water or sterile saline when there is increased potential for localized or systemic infection**.

❍ **Use sterile water delivery devices to deliver sterile solutions.** Conventional dental units cannot reliably deliver sterile water even when equipped with independent water reservoirs, because dental unit waterlines can be cleaned but not sterilized.

For more info on precautions for oral surgical procedures, see Ch. 15, which begins on p. 109.

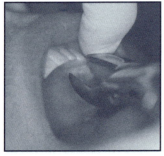

Use only sterile coolant and irrigating solutions when there is a higher risk of microorganisms gaining entry to the bloodstream, bone, or tissue under the skin.

Maintaining and Monitoring Dental Water

To ensure that water quality efforts are doing the job:

❍ Get trained on acceptable dental water quality, biofilm formation, water treatment methods, and proper maintenance protocols for water delivery systems. Treat and monitor waterline contamination as directed. Non-compliance with instructions for use has resulted in contamination in treated systems.

❍ Consult the manufacturer of your dental unit or water delivery system to find out how to best maintain treatment water quality (less than 500 CFU/mL).

❍ Monitor dental water quality at least quarterly using commercial self-contained test kits (pictured below) or commercial water-testing laboratories. This ensures that procedures are being properly performed and devices are working as they should.

In-office water testing systems work at room temperature to provide counts of bacterial colonies.

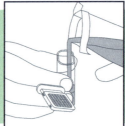 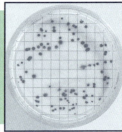

Hands-On Techniques
Monitoring Dental Water Quality

Contact the manufacturer of the dental unit and waterline maintenance system to find out the recommended monitoring schedules for the products and techniques you use. In-office test kits are available to test their dental unit water right in the office. Commercial laboratories also can test water from samples sent in by the practice. While both can be useful in managing dental water quality, laboratory tests are generally more reliable.

No matter which route you use, some general guidelines apply:

❍ If using an intermittent shock technique, test water immediately before scheduled waterline treatment.

❍ If a germicidal agent is continuously present in dental water, use a neutralizing agent if possible.

❍ Use aseptic technique to collect water samples. Pooled samples from handpieces and waterlines are acceptable except when troubleshooting units that fail to meet water quality standards. Wear clean gloves and use care not to contaminate the sample. Culture promptly following instructions for use with in-office tests or ship the sample as directed by the testing laboratory.

❍ Ensure that the laboratory is using appropriate standard methods for drinking water bacteria using lower temperature and longer incubation times.

❍ Monitor units at least quarterly and whenever starting a new waterline treatment protocol, when changing an existing waterline treatment, when new workers are given responsibility for treating dental waterlines, or after extended periods of disuse. This can be done using a water testing laboratory or in-office test kits, or a combination of the two methods.

❍ Develop and update standard operating procedures based on manufacturer instructions and train staff members on waterline maintenance and monitoring tasks.

❍ Keep records of monitoring results along with other quality assurance records such as the sterilizer monitoring log. These records should include the unit or room, date and time of sample collection, the type of test performed (in-office, laboratory), results, and methods used to correct problems including removal from service if needed.

If bacterial counts exceed 500 CFU/mL, evaluate for possible technique errors, re-treat the dental unit water, and retest. If initial testing used a pooled sample, consider testing individual lines and source water to identify the source of contamination. If a unit fails two consecutive tests, consider removing it from service and contact the manufacturer. Continue to monitor, evaluate techniques, and treat waterlines until acceptable water quality is regularly attained.

What If...

... our community is under a boil-water advisory? Can we still do dentistry?

A boil-water advisory is a notice to the public to boil tap water before drinking it. Issued by the public health department when local or regional water is deemed unsafe to drink, these advisories are issued when:

- a failure or significant interruption is detected in the municipal water treatment processes that make water safe to drink.
- pathogens such as *Cryptosporidium*, *Giardia*, or *Shigella* are discovered in the public water supply;
- the water distribution system has been compromised to the point where a health hazard exists (for example, as in a water main break);
- drinking water standards are violated for any reason; or
- natural disasters compromise quality, delivery of, or access to safe drinking water.

In the event of a boil-water advisory:

- **Do not use water from the public water supply to treat patients**. This includes water plumbed through the dental unit, ultrasonic scaler, or other equipment that uses public water. If the water source has been isolated from the municipal water system using a separate water reservoir or other water treatment device it may be possible to keep the unit in service. The unit should not be used if contaminated tap water was used to fill the reservoirs.

- **Avoid using water from faucets for patient rinsing and handwashing**. Instead:
  - Have patients rinse with bottled water.
  - For hand hygiene, use alcohol-based hand rubs if hands are not visibly soiled. If they are, use bottled water and soap or an antiseptic-containing towelette to clean the hands.

- **Treat municipal water so it is safe for hand hygiene or for diluting disinfectant chemicals** (if dilution is recommended by the germicide manufacturer):
  - Bring water to a rolling boil for at least 1 minute and cool thoroughly before use.

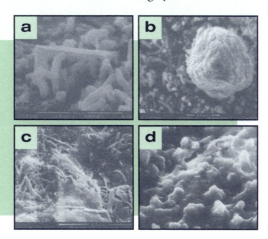

Inside dental waterlines...

(a) Microorganisms in the water attach to the tubing's inside surface, (b) form colonies, and (c) create a biofilm with (d) fully formed biofilm with protective glycocalyx (slime layer) showing complex architecture.

Boil-Water Advisory Dos and Don'ts

During a Boil-Water Advisory

DO ...

- ... Have patients use bottled water or distilled water to rinse.

- ... Use antimicrobial products that do not require water, such as alcohol-based hand rubs, for hand hygiene. If hands are visibly soiled, use bottled water and soap for handwashing or an antiseptic-containing towelette.

DON'T ...

- ... Use water from the public water system for dental treatment, patient rinsing, or handwashing.

- ... Use tap water to dilute germicides or for hand hygiene (unless the water has been brought to a rolling boil for at least 1 minute and cooled before use).

After the boil-water advisory is lifted...

DO ...

- ... Follow the local water utility's guidance for flushing all waterlines served by the public water system.

- ... Disinfect dental operative waterlines according to the manufacturer's instructions.

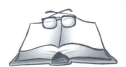

Recommended Readings and Resources

American Dental Association. Oral Health Topics. Dental Unit Waterlines Available at: *www.ada.org/en/member-center/oral-health-topics/dental-unit-waterlines*

DePaola LG, Mangan D, Mills SE, Costerton W, Barbeau J, Shearer B, Bartlett J. A review of the science regarding dental unit waterlines. *JADA* 2002;133:1199.

Kumar S, Atray D, Paiwal D, et al. Dental unit waterlines: source of contamination and cross-infection. *J Hosp Infect. 2010 Feb;74(2):99-111*

Mills S, Porteous N, Zawada J. *Dental Unit Water Quality: Organization for Safety, Asepsis and Prevention White Paper and Recommendations - 2018.* Available at: osapjdics.scholasticahq.com

Mills S. Dental Waterlines: A Decade in Review. Inside Dentistry 2006;2(3). Available at: *www.dentalaegis.com/id/2006/04/dental-waterlines-a-decade-in-review*

Mills SE. Waterborne pathogens and dental waterlines. *Dent Clin North Am* 2003;47:545.

Common Questions and Answers

Should we test our dental unit water for specific microorganisms?

Methods used to treat dental water systems target the entire biofilm, so there is usually no reason to routinely test for specific organisms such as *Legionella* or *Mycobacteria*.

What types of chemicals can we use to treat and maintain our waterlines?

The dental unit manufacturer is the best source of information on proper treatment and maintenance protocols for your dental unit, including the choice of waterline treatment agents. A number of current products use chemical agents including silver compounds, iodine, chlorhexidine gluconate and/or various oxidating agents. These agents are added to the water in the form of liquids, dissolving tablets or are slowly released from resin materials impregnated with silver compounds or iodine in either in-line cartridges connected to office plumbing or in dental water reservoir pick up tubes.

Are filters, reverse osmosis, or UV light effective in controlling water quality?

While filters, reverse osmosis systems, and UV light provide a way to improve the microbial quality of source water and are used as components of some water treatment systems, they have little or no effect on biofilm in dental unit waterlines and do not replace the use of chemical germicides to provide acceptable dental water quality.

Should we invest in a sterile water delivery system?

Sterile water delivery systems address the issue of biofilm by offering disposable or autoclavable waterline tubing that bypasses the dental unit's water supply. A number of oral-surgery handpieces, implantology handpieces, and ultrasonic scalers are equipped with their own sterile water delivery systems. Conversion kits can also provide sterile water to other instruments, such as sonic scalers and restorative handpieces.

Sterile water cannot be delivered through a standard dental unit. For practices that perform surgery with instruments that are connected to the dental unit water system, a sterile water delivery system may be a worthwhile investment. See Ch. 15, Oral Surgical Procedures, for more information.

What are the best sources of water for use in dental water reservoirs?

No dental unit can provide water that is cleaner than the water that enters it. Since units equipped with water reservoirs are filled at chairside by dental staff, aseptically introducing water with the lowest possible levels of contamination will help ensure the best results. Bottled sterile water for irrigation is an ideal source water, but cost considerations may make it impractical. Office tap water can be of acceptable quality but may become contaminated due to problems such as dead legs in office plumbing that are not reached by residual chlorine. This may also be a problem with offices that use untreated well water. Distillers and reverse osmosis systems can remove bacteria from source water, but have tubing, and storage containers can also become contaminated by biofilm and may also need to be maintained and monitored. Commercial bottled drinking water may provide a cost effective alternative, but standards for these products are not uniform and periodic testing may be prudent.

What are some of the technologies used to control dental waterline biofilm?

Products used with water reservoirs include germicidal liquids or tablets used intermittently in high concentrations (shock treatment) or slow dissolving tablets or resin impregnated pick up tubes (straws) that release low levels of biofilm control agents such as silver or iodine.

There are also devices available that use combinations of filtration, buffering and/or UV to treat water supplied by office plumbing water. These products also use slow release resins to add small quantities of germicide such as silver or iodine to control biofilm in waterlines.

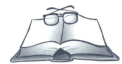

Recommended Readings and Resources

Mills SE. The dental unit waterline controversy: defusing myths, defining the solutions. *JADA* 2000; 131:1427.

Mills SE, Karpay RI. Dental waterlines and biofilm — searching for solutions. *Compend Contin Educ Dent* 2002;23:237.

OSAP. Dental Unit Waterlines Fact Sheet. Available at *www.osap.org*

OSAP. Dental Unit Waterlines – Questions and Answers. Available at *www.osap.org*

Porteous NB, Redding SW, Thompson EH, Grooters AM, De Hoog S, Sutton DA. Isolation of an unusual fungus in treated dental unit waterlines. *JADA* 2003;134:853.

Porteous NB, Partida MN. The effect of frequent clinical use of dental unit waterlines on contamination. *NY State Dent J.* 2009 Apr;75(3):20-4.

Peralta G, Tobin-D'Angelo, Parham A, et al. Notes from the Field: *Mycobacterium abscessus* Infections Among Patients of a Pediatric Dentistry Practice – *Georgia, 2015. MMWR 2016;65:355-356.*

Ricci ML, Fontana S, Pinci F et al. Pneumonia associated with a dental unit waterline. *The Lancet. 379(9816);684:2012*

Exercises in Understanding

1. Consult the owner's manual for the dental unit(s) used in your practice. What protocol(s) are recommended for controlling dental water quality?

   _____

   _____

2. What type(s) of waterline maintenance procedures are performed in your practice?

   _____

   _____

3. How often is each performed?

   _____

   _____

4. How often is dental water quality monitored, and where are the results recorded?

   _____

   _____

Self-Test

Before moving on, test yourself with some questions on the material.
(answers appear below)

1. True or False: A new dental unit will remain free of biofilm for several months.

2. During a boil-water advisory, it is acceptable to:
   a. use bottled water for patient rinsing
   b. use water from the tap but only for handwashing
   c. use an alcohol-based hand rub on soiled hands
   d. use tap water to dilute germicides as directed by the manufacturer

3. For surgical procedures:
   a. if the dental unit delivers water of less than 500 CFU/mL of bacteria, no special actions are necessary
   b. shock-treat the dental unit waterlines with a chemical agent to reduce the number of bacteria in the lines
   c. use a sterile surgical delivery system with sterile irrigating solution and coolants
   d. put sterile water for irrigation in the dental unit water reservoir instead of tap water

4. Name three types of commercially available products that can help to maintain dental water quality.

   _____ _____ _____

---

(1) False; (2) a; (3) a; (4) self-contained water systems, chemical treatments (continuous-release, intermittent, or "shock" treatments), water conditioning systems with germicidal activity, sterile water delivery systems

otes

Notes

Chapter 10

Dental Handpieces and Other Devices Attached to Air Lines and Waterlines

Examining the Issues

Several semicritical dental devices that contact mucous membranes are attached to the air lines and/or waterlines of the dental unit. These devices include:

○ highspeed and low-speed handpieces,

○ prophylaxis angles,

○ ultrasonic and sonic scaling tips,

○ air abrasion devices, and

○ air and water syringes.

These instruments have not been associated with disease transmission, but studies suggest that more stringent infection control procedures are in order.

○ Highspeed and low-speed handpieces can retract oral fluids into their internal compartments. Retracted material could later be expelled into the mouths of other patients.

○ The DNA of viruses has been found inside both highspeed handpieces and prophylaxis angles. It is not known whether the virus particles are still infectious, but their presence is a concern.

Following treatment using any dental device that enters the patient's mouth and is connected to the dental water system, run the device to discharge water, air, or a combination of both for a minimum of 20-30 seconds after each patient. This helps to physically flush out any patient material that may have entered turbines or air lines and waterlines.

For the best protection against patient-to-patient disease transmission, dental handpieces and other intraoral devices attached to air lines and/or waterlines must be sterilized using heat.

○ Neither surface disinfection nor immersion in a chemical germicide is an acceptable option for processing intraoral devices attached to air lines and/or waterlines.

Always closely follow your handpiece manufacturer's instructions for cleaning, lubrication, and sterilization to ensure both the effectiveness of the sterilization process and the longevity of handpieces. Cleaning and lubrication are most critical to handpiece performance and durability.

There are handpiece technologies in the dental market that are independent of the dental unit air and water lines. Always follow the specific handpiece manufacturer directions/instructions for reprocessing.

The Bottom Line

Because they can retract and retain patient materials, dental handpieces and other devices used in the mouth and connected to the dental unit's air lines and waterlines must be heat sterilized between patients. Components of these devices that are used outside the mouth but are prone to contamination from contact with gloves and droplet spatter should be protected with a new surface barrier for each patient and cleaned and disinfected when visibly contaminated. Always consult the owner's manual or contact the manufacturer of your handpieces and other semicritical devices for specific infection control instructions.

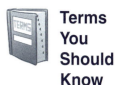

Terms You Should Know

Barrier

Cleaning

Flushing

Handpiece

Retraction

Sterilization

For definitions, see "Glossary," beginning on p. 166

Flushing the Handpiece

Flushing the handpiece after a patient visit is an important step in processing and maintenance. If debris is not removed before heat sterilization, it will bake onto the turbine and bearings. Flushing between patients is the best way to remove debris from the head of the handpiece.

Flushing a handpiece doesn't mean a quick rinse through the lines at chairside. Simply running coolant water from the dental unit through the handpiece is not sufficient. Coolant water doesn't run through the turbine chamber, where debris can collect, build up, and compromise handpiece life.

To properly flush a dental handpiece:

1 Attach a pressurized handpiece cleaner to the intake tube of the handpiece and flush the head of the handpiece — where the air passes through — with the cleaner to remove debris.

2 Afterward, blow out the handpiece using compressed air to remove debris and cleaner before sterilization.

Your handpiece manufacturer can recommend a suitable cleaner.

NOTE: Most handpieces should not be run without a bur in place. Consult the user's guide of your handpiece for proper procedures.

Patient Safety and Devices Connected to the Dental Unit

To ensure the safest environment for your patients...

In the operatory ...

○ **Only use disposable or heat-tolerant devices that are connected to the dental unit** for use in the patient's mouth (see Ch. 13, Single-Use [Disposable] Devices).

○ **Use fluid-proof surface barriers to cover dental instrument components that do not enter the patient's mouth, are not removable, and are likely to become contaminated** during treatment procedures. Examples include handles or dental unit attachments of saliva ejectors, high-speed air evacuators, and air-water syringes. If these instrument surfaces become visibly contaminated during use, clean them and use an intermediate-level disinfectant before using them on the next patient. Follow instructions for contact time on the disinfectant's label.

During processing ...

○ **Always follow the manufacturer's instructions for between-patient cleaning, lubricating, and heat sterilizing** handpieces and other intraoral instruments that can be removed from the air lines and waterlines of dental units.

○ **Between patients, thoroughly clean and heat sterilize contaminated handpieces and other intraoral instruments** that can be removed from the air lines and waterlines of dental units. See "Step-by-Step: Handpiece Processing" (next page) for an overview of procedures.

  ❐ **Unless they will be used immediately after sterilization, package handpieces and other devices** in bags, wraps, or packs compatible with the sterilization method. This protects them from contamination after the cycle and before use at chairside.

  ❐ **Use an autoclave or chemical vapor sterilizer to process handpieces** at a temperature of approximately 275°F/135°C. The high temperatures (325°F/163°C) and long cycle times used by dry heat sterilizers are inappropriate for handpieces and can cause irreversible damage. Follow the handpiece manufacturer's instructions for the method of sterilization as well as for cycle time and temperature.

  ❐ **Immediate use sterilization** (formerly called flash sterilization) of single, unwrapped instruments is appropriate only when presented with an urgent need to sterilize a particular instrument (for example, your only handpiece fell to the floor during treatment). For more information on immediate use sterilization, see p. 51.

○ **Process devices connected to the dental unit and used in the mouth along with other heat-tolerant instruments and patient-care items**. A special cycle is not required.

○ **Do not use surface disinfectants, liquid chemical sterilants, or ethylene oxide on handpieces**. (Chemical germicides and ethylene oxide gas cannot adequately sterilize the components inside the handpiece.)

Cleaning and lubrication are the most critical factors in determining handpiece performance and durability.

Closely follow the handpiece manufacturer's instructions for cleaning, lubricating, and heat sterilizing to ensure the effectiveness of the sterilization process and the longevity of your handpieces. Failure to do so can void a handpiece's warranty.

Step by Step

Handpiece Processing: General Recommendations

NOTE: This protocol represents typical handpiece preparation and processing procedures for handpieces that are rated as "sterilizable" by the manufacturer. It is intended only to provide an overview of general procedures. Always follow the handpiece manufacturer's instructions for maintenance and sterilization. Failure to do so can void the handpiece's warranty.

1 Before removing the handpiece from the hose after treatment, with the bur still in the chuck, briefly run the water/air system to flush waterlines and air lines.

2 Remove the bur from the handpiece, wipe visible debris from the outer surfaces of the handpiece, and disconnect the handpiece from the hose.
- ❍ If ultrasonic cleaning is deemed acceptable by the handpiece manufacturer, follow instructions to ultrasonically clean the handpiece head or the entire handpiece, then thoroughly drain the instrument, attach the hose, and briefly operate the handpiece to expel debris.
- ❍ If ultrasonic cleaning is not expressly stated as acceptable, scrub the handpiece thoroughly under running water with a brush and soap/detergent cleaner.

3 If the handpiece requires lubrication before heat-processing, use a handpiece cleaner recommended by the manufacturer that will both remove internal debris and lubricate the handpiece. See p. 84, "Flushing the Handpiece," for more info on cleaning and flushing.
- ❍ If the handpiece does not require lubrication before processing, use a cleaner that does not contain a lubricant.
- ❍ Follow the manufacturer's instructions for each type of handpiece used.
- ❍ Do not overlubricate handpieces.

4 Reattach the handpiece to a hose and operate the drive air system to blow excess lubricant from the rotating parts. Failure to perform this step before heat sterilization can lead to excess lubricant accumulation in the working assembly and "gumming" in the rotating assemblies during the heat cycle.

— or —

As an alternative to reattaching the handpiece to the hose, for systems with directly accessible drive air tubes, use an air-water syringe to blow into the drive air tube on the back end of the handpiece (usually the shorter/smaller of the two larger tubes).

— or —

Use an automated cleaner/lubricator or air station to flush the handpiece.

NOTE: Most handpieces should not be run without a bur or bur blank in the chuck. Be sure to check with the handpiece manufacturer before attempting no-load operation.

NOTE: Do not lubricate handpieces in the operatory. This task is best performed on the "dirty" side of the instrument processing area (see Ch. 7, Sterilization and Disinfection of Patient-Care Items).

5 Using a cotton swab dampened (not soaked) with isopropyl alcohol, remove all excess lubricant from fiberoptic interfaces and exposed optical surfaces.
- ❍ Never use strong solvents on fiberoptic interfaces. They can dissolve the epoxy binder between the fibers.

continued on next page

Handpiece Processing

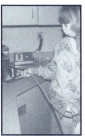 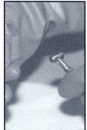

After treatment, run the air and water system, then remove the bur from the chuck.

Wipe debris from the handpiece surface, and disconnect it from the hose.

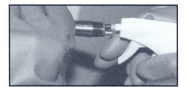

Flush the handpiece according to the manufacturer's recommendations. If lubrication is required, use a combination cleaner-lubricant.

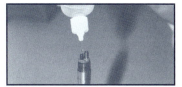

If the manufacturer recommends a separate lubricant, use only a few drops. Overlubricating can hamper sterilization and slow turbines.

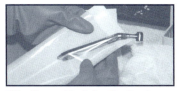

After thoroughly drying the handpiece, package it for sterilization.

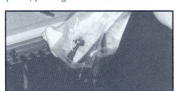

After the cycle when the handpiece has cooled down and is about to be used, open the sterile pack at chairside to show the patient that the instrument has been sterilized.

Get a Handle on Contamination Control

While the handles and controls of devices used in the mouth never actually enter the oral cavity, they are prone to contamination from contact with gloved hands and droplet spatter. These surfaces are often very difficult to clean.

Use impervious barriers to cover dental instrument components that do not enter the patient's mouth but are likely to become contaminated during treatment procedures. Change these barriers after each use. Such parts include but are not limited to the handles or dental unit attachments of:

○ saliva ejectors,
○ highspeed air evacuators,
○ air-water syringes, and
○ curing lights.

If controls or handles become visibly contaminated during use, clean and intermediate-level disinfect them before use on the next patient. Follow instructions for contact time on the disinfectant's label.

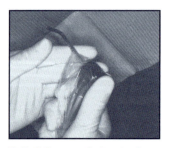

To limit the spread of contamination to difficult-to-clean surfaces such as buttons and knobs, barrier-protect handles and controls of devices that are used in the mouth.

Step by Step

Handpiece processing *continued from p. 85*

6 Make sure the handpiece is clean, then dry it internally and externally and package it for sterilization. Sterilize according to the sterilizer and handpiece manufacturers' instructions. After the heat cycle, allow the bagged handpiece to cool and dry. Keep sterilization packaging sealed until the handpiece is to be prepared for use on a patient.

7 Flush waterlines and air lines of the handpiece hose for 20 to 30 seconds before attaching the handpiece.

8 If the handpiece does not require post-sterilization lubrication:
○ Open the sterilization bag at chairside in front of the patient to demonstrate that a fresh instrument is being used.

If handpiece requires post-sterilization lubrication:
○ Reserve a separate lubricant canister for post-cycle use and lubricate the handpiece as close to the actual time of use as feasible. This reduces the chance of cross-contamination.
  ❏ Open just the end of the sterilization packaging and spray the lubricant into the handpiece air drive tube to reduce the amount of overspray and help control excess lubricant.
NOTE: A handpiece that requires post-sterilization lubrication cannot be used for oral surgical procedures. It is no longer sterile.

! **The handpiece is now ready for use.**

Extending Handpiece Life

The average life of a highspeed dental handpiece has been estimated at 8 to 14 months, although life expectancy can vary widely depending on patient volume, conditions of use, and maintenance.

Here are some tips for extending the life of your handpiece without compromising patient safety.

○ Always follow the manufacturer's specific instructions for maintaining each brand/type of handpiece.
  ❏ Keep instructions on maintenance procedures handy.
  ❏ Take part in in-service training in your practice setting, whether you're a new or experienced dental worker. Different brands of handpieces can have different maintenance protocols, so be sure your procedures are right for the handpiece. "Refresher" training also is helpful — perhaps every 3 months — to ensure that proper procedures remain in practice.
○ If you are responsible for preparing handpieces for sterilization, make sure you have the time and facilities to do the job. If you find yourself tempted to take shortcuts because of time constraints, speak with your employer or Infection Control Coordinator. Shortcuts can compromise both patient safety and handpiece life.
○ Routinely service handpieces before they fail. Set up a schedule to rotate handpieces back to the manufacturer for refurbishing. Scheduling such service during vacations or over holidays makes sure the practice won't be short of instruments.

Common Questions and Answers

Why do handpieces fail? Is it because of the sterilization cycle?

While the highspeed handpieces available in most parts of the world today are heat-tolerant, they have a definite use life and require periodic maintenance for proper operation. The most common causes of handpiece failure are debris and overheating, which are more closely associated with inadequate cleaning than with the heat sterilization process.

Debris can enter the handpiece through contaminated air and water, or through retraction. It's important to always use a clean, oil-free air supply. As the handpiece operates, air passes over the turbine to make it spin. If there is debris in the air, it can collect on the turbine and the turbine head. From there it can work its way up into the bearings, where it will cause the handpiece to fail. Likewise, when the handpiece is shut down, air pressure is released and an air vacuum results. This vacuum can pull debris such as blood, tooth fragments, and saliva from the patient's mouth into the head of the handpiece.

If debris is not removed prior to heat sterilization, it will bake onto the turbine and bearings. Flushing the handpiece head (see p. 84) between patients with a manufacturer-recommended cleaner is the best way to remove debris.

What type of sterilizer should we use for our highspeed handpieces?

Because handpiece sterilization temperatures should not exceed 275°F/135°C, currently only autoclaves and chemical-vapor sterilizers are recommended depending on the manufacturer's directions. Most full-size sterilizers complete their cycles and deliver bagged, dry instruments within an hour.

Immediate use sterilization (formerly called flash sterilization) where instruments are sterilized unpackaged, should be avoided. Also, the high temperatures (325°F/163°C) and long cycle times used in dry heat sterilization are not compatible with dental handpieces.

Should we lubricate our handpieces?

Not all highspeed handpieces require lubrication. Different handpiece manufacturers have different maintenance requirements. Always follow the instructions outlined by the manufacturer of your handpiece.

If a separate lubricant is recommended, be sure to hook up the handpiece to a proper air supply and expel any excess prior to sterilization.

Avoid over-lubricating the handpiece. Introduced prior to the heat cycle, too much lubrication can hinder the sterilization process. The sterilizing agent must contact all surfaces to ensure sterility, and oils can act as a barrier between instruments and the sterilizing agent. In addition, excess lubricant can cause a tar-like residue to build up in the bearings, which results in slowing and loss of power of the handpiece. Added after sterilization, over-lubrication hinders handpiece performance, because its extra mass slows turbines.

Did You Know...?

... the real story on saliva ejectors?

During World War I, the warning was that "Loose lips sink ships." In the dental operatory, however, loose lips prevent oral fluids from retracting into your devices, air lines, and waterlines.

Suctioned fluids can be pulled into the patient's mouth when a seal around the saliva ejector is created, such as when the patient closes his or her lips around the tip of the ejector.

Don't ask your patients to close their lips around the saliva ejector tip. Although there appear to be no reports of illness associated with saliva ejectors, limiting contamination and in turn, the risk for disease transmission, is a basic principle of infection control.

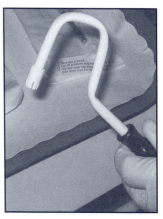

Don't ask patients to close their lips around a saliva ejector. Doing so creates a seal that can cause suctioned fluids to retract into the patient's mouth.

To Extend the Life of Your Handpiece...

Before use:

◯ Ensure that the air supply is dry and debris-free

◯ Ensure that the water supply is debris-free

◯ Ensure that air pressure is under 40 psi, unless otherwise advised by the manufacturer

◯ Ensure that the handpiece is at room temperature after sterilization

During use:

◯ Keep air pressure under 40 psi

◯ Try not to use long or large-head burs

◯ With pushbutton spindles, do not use under- or over-sized burs

◯ Don't use highspeed handpieces in the dental lab

After use on a patient:

◯ Flush the handpiece with a handpiece cleaner before sterilization

◯ Ensure that the sterilizer does not exceed 275°F/135°C

◯ Do not leave handpieces in the sterilizer overnight

◯ If directed to lubricate after sterilization, use just a few drops of oil

Weekly maintenance:

◯ Flush pushbutton spindles with a handpiece cleaner

Quarterly maintenance:

◯ Check any air and water supply filters and dryers

Turbine replacements:

◯ Ultrasonically clean the handpiece shell before installation

◯ Flush handpiece shell and clean head after ultrasonic cleaner use

◯ Replace O-rings, springs, washers, and clips

Exercises in Understanding

1. Which devices connected to the dental unit in your operatories are used in the mouth? How is each processed between patients?

Device	Processed by...

2. How are the handles, attachments, and connectors of each of these devices protected from cross-contamination (for example, with a surface cover or between-patient cleaning and disinfection)?

Device	Protected by...

3. What method of heat sterilization is used in your practice setting to sterilize highspeed and low-speed handpieces?

_____

What cycle time and temperature is used?

Cycle time: _____   Cycle temperature: _____

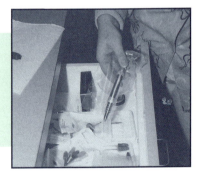

If they will not be used immediately, store sterile handpiece packs in drawers or cabinets to reduce the chance of contamination.

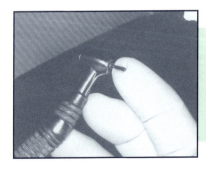

Always use care when handling burs. They are sharp cutting instruments, and they can cause injury.

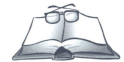

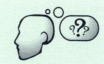

What If...

...we need to use our handpiece as soon as it comes out of the sterilizer? Can we cool it by running sterile water over it?

Never run a handpiece hot out of the sterilizer, and avoid rapid cool-downs, such as running the hot handpiece under cold water.

Handpieces use very small metal components. Taking the devices from very hot to very cold puts a lot of stress on the metal.

If you find that you routinely don't have enough time to cool handpieces before they are needed, encourage your employer or office manager to consider purchasing additional handpieces.

Self-Test

Before moving on, test yourself with some questions on the material.
(answers appear below)

1. Always run highspeed handpieces when they are:
   a. hot out of the sterilizer
   b. at room temperature
   c. cooled under cold running water
   d. any of the above

2. The most important factor(s) in handpiece performance and life is (are):
   a. sterilization temperature
   b. packaging materials and cycle times
   c. cleaning and lubrication
   d. the germicide used to disinfect it

3. True or False: Always ask your patients to close their lips around the saliva ejector tip.

4. A highspeed handpiece is a _____ instrument and should be processed using _____.
   a. critical ... heat sterilization
   b. semicritical ... high-level disinfection
   c. semicritical ... heat sterilization
   d. semicritical ... surface disinfection

5. Which of the following may be used to process handpieces for use on the next patient?
   a. autoclave
   b. ethylene oxide
   c. liquid chemical sterilant
   d. dry heat

Recommended Readings and Resources

American Dental Association. Sterilization and Disinfection of Dental Instruments. Updated July 2009. Available at: *www.ada.org/~/media/ADA/Member%20Center/FIles/cdc_sterilization.ashx*

Centers for Disease Control and Prevention. Healthcare Infection Control Practices Advisory Committee (HICPAC). Guideline for Disinfection and Sterilization in Healthcare Facilities, 2008. Dental Instruments. Available at: *www.cdc.gov/hicpac/Disinfection_Sterilization/3_1deLaparoArthro.html*

Barbeau J, ten Bokum L, Gauthier C, Prevost AP. Cross-contamination potential of saliva ejectors used in dentistry. *J Hosp Infect* 1998;40:303.

Epstein JB, Rea G, Sibau L, Sherlock CH, Le ND. Assessing viral retention and elimination in rotary dental instruments. *JADA* 1995;126:87.

Kuehne JS, Cohen ME, Monreo SB. Performance and durability of autoclavable high speed handpieces. *Naval Dent Res Inst PR* 1992;(May):92.

Leonard DL, Charlton DG. Performance of high-speed dental handpieces subjected to simulated clinical use and sterilization. *JADA* 1999;130:1301.

(1) b; (2) c; (3) False; (4) c; (5) a.

Notes

Dental Radiography

Examining the Issues

Although no direct evidence suggests that a disease can be transmitted via dental x-ray procedures, the activities surrounding taking x-rays offer many chances for spreading germs. Digital x-ray sensors and film packets used in the mouth are contaminated, touched and then transported to another part of the facility. Any time something comes in contact with digital sensors or x-ray film packets that were used in a patient's mouth, it becomes contaminated. Similarly, all surfaces touched during x-ray procedures can become contaminated, including clinical contact surfaces such as computer keyboard/mouse, x-ray sensor cords, and portable equipment carts.

Radiographic equipment can become contaminated when x-rays are taken, and film processing equipment contaminated when x-ray film is developed. Oral microorganisms can survive on radiographic equipment for at least 48 hours and can remain alive in developer/fixer for up to two weeks. Even without films or processing equipment, digital x-rays bring their own infection control challenges. Although they are semicritical instruments, the sensors used in the mouth to take filmless x-rays may not be heat-tolerant or able to withstand soaking in a chemical sterilant.

For infection control during radiographic procedures:

❍ Disposable and heat-sterilizable x-ray accessories such as bite guides, film holders, and film positioning devices help to limit the spread of contamination between patients. Discard disposable devices after use on one patient; heat sterilize heat-tolerant accessories between patient uses. For semicritical items that cannot be heat sterilized, use a liquid chemical sterilant/high-level disinfectant.

❍ Heat-sensitive x-ray sensors that are used in the mouth but cannot be heat sterilized or soaked in a liquid chemical disinfectant should be barrier protected during use. After use, clean and intermediate-level disinfect them according to the device manufacturer's instructions. Digital x-ray sensors are semicritical items.

❍ Surface covers can protect clinical contact surfaces from contamination. Uncovered equipment surfaces and controls that are touched during dental x-ray procedures must be cleaned and disinfected between patients.

The Bottom Line

Infection control practices for dental radiology are identical to those used in the operatory. They are based on standard precautions and are aimed at preventing disease transmission from patient to dental worker, from dental worker to patient, and from patient to patient.

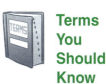

Terms You Should Know

Barrier

Clinical contact surface

Cross-contamination

High-level disinfectant

Intermediate-level disinfectant

Semicritical instrument

Standard precautions

Sterilization

For definitions, see "Glossary," *beginning on p. 166*

Did You Know ...

... that a lot of surfaces can easily become contaminated when taking and developing dental x-rays?

Any surfaces that you touch or that you lay contaminated items upon become contaminated, including:

○ tubehead
○ extension cone
○ control panel
○ exposure button
○ chair/headrest controls
○ darkroom
○ processors
○ any environmental surfaces contacted by gloved hands, contaminated film packets, or devices used in the mouth

Use barriers to protect surfaces that are prone to contamination, shorten turnaround time between patients, and reduce the need for disinfectants that can damage surfaces and linger in the air.

○ **Cover surfaces/objects that may be touched with contaminated hands or contaminated objects**.

○ **Use disposable, fluid-proof materials**

○ **Change barriers between patients** — it only takes a few seconds!

Step by Step

Standard Intraoral X-rays

Before taking the x-rays...

1 Use disposable or heat-tolerant versions of intraoral x-ray accessories when available. Heat-sterilize reusable, heat-tolerant devices before use.

2 Protect radiography equipment (such as the x-ray tubehead and control panel) with clean surface barriers.

3 Unit-dose all necessary supplies, equipment, and instruments prior to patient seating. Aseptically dispense film from the central supply area into a clean disposable container.

4 Have the patient rinse with a preprocedural mouthrinse, if desired (see Ch. 14, Preprocedural Mouthrinsing).

5 Provide the patient with a lead apron with thyroid collar to protect against any scatter radiation.

6 Wash hands, dry thoroughly, and put on exam gloves.

While taking the x-rays...

7 Wear gloves when taking radiographs and handling contaminated film packets. Wear other personal protective equipment (e.g., face shield, surgical mask, protective eyewear, gowns) if spatter is likely (see Ch. 5, Personal Protective Equipment, for more info).

8 Touch as few surfaces as possible.

9 Stay behind the protective lead partition until after the exposure.

10 Following exposure of the radiograph, with gloves still in place, dry the film with disposable gauze or a paper towel to remove blood or excess saliva.

11 Drop the film packet into a container (such as a paper or plastic cup). Be careful not to contaminate the outside of the container.

12 Repeat until the x-ray series is complete.

After taking the x-rays...

13 Place reusable film-holding devices in the designated area.

14 If film barrier pouches have been used, carefully peel back the barrier and allow each film packet to fall from its pouch into a clean disposable container (such as a plastic cup) for transport to the developing area.
   ○ Use care to avoid contaminating the outside of the film packet and the cup.
   If barrier pouches have not been used, follow instructions on the next page for "Handling Film Without Barriers."

15 Discard all contaminated disposable items.

16 Carefully remove contaminated barriers from covered surfaces.

17 Remove gloves and wash hands.

18 Remove the lead apron and dismiss the patient.

19 Disinfect all uncovered surfaces that were contaminated.
 ○ If barriers are not used, x-ray equipment that has come into contact with gloved hands or contaminated film packets must be cleaned and then disinfected after each patient. Use a low- (with HIV and HBV claim) to intermediate-level (tuberculocidal activity) hospital disinfectant registered with the Environmental Protection Agency (EPA).

For developing film...

20 With clean, ungloved hands, transport the disposable container of exposed film to the processing area.

21 Unit dose:
 ○ gloves
 ○ paper towel(s)
 ○ paper cup(s)
 ○ film mount or paper envelope

22 Take care to avoid contaminating the developing equipment.
 ○ Use protective barriers or clean and disinfect any contaminated surfaces by using an EPA-registered low- (with HIV and HBV claim) to intermediate-level (tuberculocidal activity) hospital disinfectant.

Handling Film Without Barrier Pouches

Barrier sleeves for x-ray film packets are commercially available. These barriers are placed over the x-ray film packet before the film is positioned in the patient's mouth and removed immediately after the x-ray is taken, providing dental workers with a clean, uncontaminated film packet for processing.

The barriers protect film from contamination, reduce preparation time, and simplify processing. Removed in a lighted area with gloved hands, the barrier is peeled back and the film packet dropped onto a clean paper towel or into a clean disposable cup. Barrier-protected film packs are especially useful when using a daylight loader (p. 94).

If your practice setting uses film that is not barrier-protected, add these steps to the infection control protocol for dental x-rays:

a	Place paper towel	**g**	Allow film to drop onto paper towel
b	Place container with films next to paper towel	**h**	Dispose of empty packet
c	Secure door and turn out light (if applicable)	**i**	After all film packets have been opened, discard container
d	Put on gloves	**j**	Remove gloves and wash hands
e	Remove film from container	**k**	Process film by edges only
f	Open film packet	**l**	Label film mount or envelope

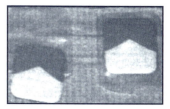

Use barriers to protect x-ray film from contamination, reduce preparation time, and simplify processing.

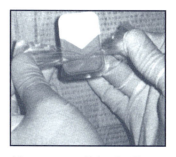

After exposure, with hands still gloved, carefully peel back the barrier (above). Allow each film packet to fall from its pouch into a clean, disposable cup.

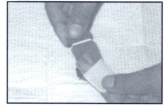

Once in the processing area, open the film packet with clean, ungloved hands.

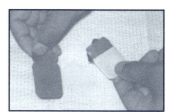

Holding the tab, gently drop the film onto a clean surface.

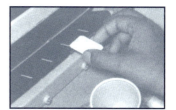

Holding the film by the edges, insert it into the processor.

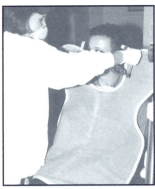

To protect against scatter radiation, give your patients a lead apron and thyroid collar when taking dental x-rays.

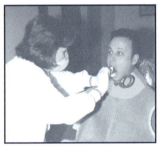

Because they contact mucous membranes, x-ray positioning guides are semicritical instruments. If they are heat-tolerant, sterilize them using heat. If not, use a chemical sterilant/high-level disinfectant.

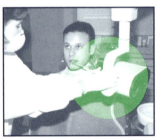

The x-ray tubehead is a clinical contact surface. In the practice setting shown above, it must be cleaned and disinfected before the next patient. Use a surface barrier to save turnaround time.

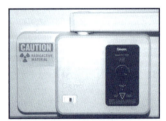

Dental x-ray machines use radiation. Exposure to radiation can cause cancer. X-rays cannot penetrate lead, so always stay behind the protective lead partition until after the exposure.

Step by Step

Panoramic/Cephalometric X-rays

Few intraoral components are involved in panoramic and cephalometric x-rays, so infection control is simplified.

1 Wash hands prior to taking extraoral film.

2 Barrier-protect bite guides. Disposable and reusable heat-tolerant bite guides provide other options.

3 Consider barriers for the chin rest, head positioning guides, and hand grips.

4 Handle extraoral cassettes with ungloved hands.

5 After x-ray exposure, have the patient remove the barrier from the bite guide and discard it in the regular office trash bin.

Step by Step

Using a Daylight Loader for Processing Dental X-ray Film

Because they have cloth or rubber sleeves, cuffs, or flaps to allow access to the x-ray processing chamber without allowing light exposure, daylight loaders present additional infection control challenges.

1 With clean hands, open the lid of the loader and place a paper towel, paper cup, and powder-free gloves inside the loader's compartment.

2 Place container with contaminated films next to the paper cup.

3 Close the lid and place hands through the sleeves and into the compartment.

4 Put on clean gloves.

5 Remove one film from the container, and open packet as previously described.

6 Allow film to drop onto paper towel or processor film feed slot.

7 Dispose of film packet contents in empty paper cup.

8 Repeat until all packets have been opened.

9 After opening all packets, remove gloves and place them in the cup.

10 Feed all films into the processor, handling them only by the edges.

11 Remove hands from the loader.

12 Wash and dry hands.

13 Lift the lid to the loader compartment and remove all contents.

14 Label film mount or paper envelope.

Common Questions and Answers

Our x-ray positioners can't be autoclaved. How do we process them?

X-ray positioners, film holders, and other devices used in the mouth in dental radiography are semicritical instruments. That is, they contact only intact mucous membranes. Although heat-tolerant or single-use disposable intraoral devices are preferred for this application, reusable semi-critical heat-sensitive devices can be cleaned and then chemically sterilized/high-level disinfected before use on the next patient.

We use digital x-rays and the sensors can't be cleaned. How can we make them safe for use from one patient to the next?

Digital radiography sensors and other "high-tech" instruments such as intraoral cameras, electronic periodontal probes, occlusal analyzers, and dental and soft tissue lasers are semicritical devices. They contact mucous membranes.

Of course, heat sterilization is preferred for all semi-critical instruments. Although these devices cannot withstand heat or chemical immersion, most digital x-ray sensors can be cleaned and disinfected. Cover such devices with a surface barrier during patient use. Protective sheaths are commercially available for many intraoral components of high-tech equipment. Barriers that are designed for handpieces and air-water syringes and are closed on one end also may work well. Digital x-ray sensors with cords can be covered using a longer plastic sleeve that protects both the device and its cord.

Barriers can help eliminate gross contamination on devices used in the mouth, but they do not always protect from all possible contamination. Because the device will be reused in another patient's mouth, cleaning and intermediate-level disinfection is recommended after the barrier is removed. Wipe sensors with a disinfectant-soaked gauze pad or a disinfectant wipe.

Consult your high-tech device's user's manual for complete infection control instructions.

Managing Semicritical X-ray Devices

If the Device...			
Cannot Be Cleaned	**Can Be Cleaned and Is...**		
	Heat-tolerant	**Not heat-tolerant**	**Not heat-tolerant and can't be immersed**
Barrier protect during patient use and change barriers between patients	Clean and then heat-sterilize between patients	Clean and then high-level disinfect between patients	Barrier protect during patient use; change barriers between patients After treatment of each patient, remove the barrier, then clean and disinfect the device using an intermediate-level surface disinfectant

-Minimizing Contamination

To reduce the spread of contamination, and in turn, the risk of disease transmission during dental x-ray procedures:

❍ Wash your hands

❍ Use personal protective equipment

❍ Use surface barriers

❍ Clean or disinfect equipment surfaces that are not covered

❍ Clean and heat sterilize instruments and items used to take dental radiographs

❍ Unit-dose the supplies you will need before seating the patient

Unit-dosing minimizes cross-contamination, saves chairside time, and reduces worker contact with surfaces.

To prepare for a patient appointment involving dental radiography, unit-dose the following:

❍ Paper towels

❍ Surface disinfectant

❍ Surface barriers

❍ Powder-free gloves

❍ X-ray film(s)

❍ Sterile or disposable film holders

❍ Paper cups or plastic bags

❍ Lead apron with thyroid collar

❍ Cotton rolls (to stabilize film placement and remove saliva from film)

❍ Preprocedural mouthrinse, if desired (see Ch. 14, Preprocedural Mouthrinsing)

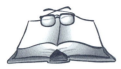

Recommended Readings and Resources

Bartoloni JA, Charlton DG, Flint DJ. Infection control practices in dental radiology. *Gen Dent* 2003;51:264.

Hubar JS, Gardiner DM. Infection control procedures used in conjunction with computed dental radiography. *Int J Comput Dent* 2000 Oct;3(4):259.

Hokett SD, Honey JR, Ruiz F, Baisden MK, Hoen MM. Assessing the effectiveness of direct digital radiography barrier sheaths and finger cots. *JADA* 2000;131:463.

Wenzel A, Frandsen E, Hintze H. Patient discomfort and cross-infection control in bitewing examination with a storage phosphor plate and a CCD-based sensor. *J Dent* 1999;27:243.

Puttaiah R, Langlais RP, Katz JO, Langland OE. Infection control in dental radiology. *W V Dent J* 1995 Jun;69(3):15.

Wyche CJ. Infection control protocols for exposing and processing radiographs. *J Dent Hyg* 1996 May-Jun;70(3):122.

Exercises in Understanding

Work with a coworker or your Infection Control Coordinator. Walk through a typical patient seating for dental x-rays. How many opportunities for contamination can you identify? How does your practice control contamination in each situation (for example, by placing surface barriers, using personal protective equipment, disinfecting or sterilizing items, etc.)?

Action and surface that becomes contaminated	Action to prevent, limit, control or manage contamination

Self-Test

Before moving on, test yourself with some questions on the material.
(answers appear below)

1. Why do daylight loaders present an additional infection control challenge?
   _____

2. Manage contamination of heat-sensitive semicritical instruments that cannot be soaked in liquid by:
   a. barrier protecting during use
   b. cleaning then disinfecting with an intermediate-level disinfectant after treatment
   c. wiping down with glutaraldehyde
   d. both a and b

3. Name three clinical contact surfaces involved in taking a dental x-ray.
   _____ _____ _____

4. True or False: The radiation used in a dental x-ray is not at all hazardous; no safety precautions are required.

(1) Because they have cloth or rubber sleeves, cuffs, or flaps. (2) d; (3) tubehead, extension cone, control panel, exposure button, chair/headrest controls, any other environmental surfaces contacted by gloved hands, contaminated film packets, or devices used in the mouth; (4) False

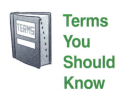

Chapter 12

Aseptic Technique for Parenteral Medications

Examining the Issues

When needles pierce the skin or mucous membranes during the delivery of intravenous (IV) medications, local anesthetics or other drugs, there is a risk of infectious disease transmission or needlestick injury. Safe injection practices, an important part of standard precautions, aim to prevent such transmissions or injuries and maintain basic levels of patient safety and clinician protection. Safe injection practices became part of standard precautions in 2007. However, some aspects of safe injection practices were included in CDC's 2003 dental infection control guidelines as recommendations for using aseptic technique for parenteral medications.

Parenteral medications - those that are injected or administered by intravenous (IV) catheter - break the skin barrier. This means that contaminated medications, needles and syringes present a higher risk of bloodborne disease transmission. As such aseptic technique (actions that limit contamination) is extremely important when handling and delivering these medications to patients. Outbreaks of hepatitis B and C have been traced to needles that were reused on multiple patients and to medication vials that were contaminated by used needles.

Parenteral medications may be supplied in single-use or multiple-dose packaging.
○ Single-dose ampules, vials, or pre-filled syringes are intended for use on only one patient. They contain no preservatives.
○ Multiple-dose vials, used several times for one or more patients, may contain a preservative.

Both single-use and multiple-dose containers of parenteral medications can become contaminated, creating a risk of infection and disease transmission.
○ When used on just one patient with a sterile needle, single-dose medication vials are the safer option. However, even single-dose vials can become contaminated if they are punctured several times. Because of this, never use single-dose parenteral medications on more than one patient.
○ If a needle that has been used on a patient draws from a multiple-dose vial, bloodborne and other pathogens from the patient can be introduced to the vial, then spread to the next patient who is injected with medication from the vial.

To limit contamination, store and prepare injectable medications in a central medication preparation area that is separate from the treatment area.

See Appendix A for CDC's recommendations for Safe Injection Practices and for Aseptic Technique for Parenteral Medications.

Terms You Should Know

Aseptic technique

Bloodborne disease(s)

Conscious sedation

Cross-contamination

Fluid infusion system

Healthcare-associated infection

IV catheter

Parenteral

Parenteral medication

For definitions, see "Glossary," *beginning on page 166*

The Bottom Line

Whether using single-use or multi-dose containers, always use aseptic techniques to prevent contamination of parenteral medication.

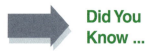

Did You Know ...

... that both the needle and syringe used to access a multiple-dose vial must be sterile?

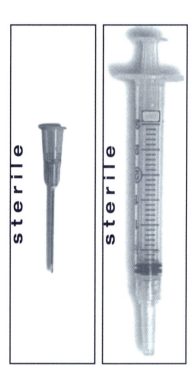

sterile

sterile

! Never reuse a syringe even if the needle is changed.

! Whenever possible, use single-dose vials for parenteral medications.

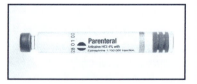

Used for only one patient, single-dose parenteral medication cartridges greatly reduce the risk of disease transmission.

Safe Injection Practices

As with all aspects of dental infection control, the key to injection safety is limiting contamination.

Always ... !

○ **Always use aseptic technique in a clean area when preparing injections or IV equipment.**
   ❑ Wear gloves and use care to prevent cross-contamination.
   ❑ Wipe the access diaphragm of a medication vial with alcohol to disinfect.

○ **Always choose and use single-dose vials when available.**

○ **Always discard single-use vials after use, including any leftover contents.**

○ **Always try to dedicate multi-dose vials to a single patient.**
   ❑ If you intended to use multi-dose vials for more than one patient:
      • keep the vials in a centralized area away from the patient treatment area to prevent contamination. If a multi-dose vial is brought into the patient treatment area dedicate it for that single patient and discard immediately after use.

○ **Always write the current date on the multi-dose vial and discard within 28 days** unless the manufacturer specifies a shorter or longer time for discard.

○ **Always discard a multiple-dose vial** if sterility is compromised.

○ **Always treat all IV bags and connections as single-patient, disposable items.** Sterility cannot be guaranteed when an infusion or administration set is used on multiple patients.

Never ... !

○ **Never reuse needles or syringes to enter a medication vial or solution,** even when obtaining additional doses for the same patient.

○ **Never use single-dose (single-use)** medication vials, amuples, and bags or bottles of intravenous solution for more than one patient.

○ **Never combine medications left in an ampule or vial** with other medications for use on another patient.

○ **Never administer medication from a syringe to multiple patients**, even if the needle on the syringe is changed.

○ **Never carry medication vials, syringes, or supplies in pockets of your uniform** or clothing.

○ **Never use fluid infusion and administration sets** (IV bags and connections) **for more than one patient**. IV bag and connections cannot be adequately cleaned and sterilized.

If ... then ... !

○ **If the sterility of a multiple-dose vial has been compromised, then discard the vial** and any remaining contents.

○ **If trays are used to deliver medications to individual patients, then clean the trays between patients** to prevent cross-contamination.

○ **If you must use a multiple-dose vial, then:**
   ❑ **cleanse the access diaphragm with 70% alcohol** before inserting a sterile needle or other device into the vial,
   ❑ **use a sterile device to access the vial**, and
   ❑ **avoid touching the access diaphragm**.

Exercises in Understanding

1. If parenteral medications are utilized in your clinic setting, what type of dispenser(s) are used?

   Single use? _____

   Multiple-dose? _____

   Both? _____

2. Where are parenteral medications stored in your practice?

   _____

3. Are parenteral medications stored away from the operatory and safe from contamination? If not, where could they be stored to better protect them from contact and droplet contamination?

   _____

Self-Test

Before moving on, test yourself with some questions on the material.
(answers appear below)

1. True or False: Only multiple-dose vials of parenteral medications are at risk of being contaminated.

2. True or False: It is okay to administer medication from one syringe to multiple patients as long as the needle is changed.

3. Always or Never: _____ reuse IV sets.

4. Always or Never: _____ choose single-dose packaging over multiple-dose packaging for parenteral medications.

5. Always or Never: _____ combine medications leftover in a single-use ampule to save money.

6. Always or Never: _____ carry an extra ampule of anesthetic in your uniform pocket to save time.

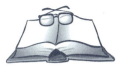

Recommended Readings and Resources

Centers for Disease Control and Prevention. Transmission of Hepatitis B and C Viruses in Outpatient Settings — New York, Oklahoma, and Nebraska, 2000-2002. *MMWR Morbid Mortal Weekly Report* 2003; 52(38):901.

Centers for Disease Control and Prevention. Injection Safety, Information for Providers: Available at: *www.cdc.gov/injection safety/*

Centers for Disease Control and Prevention. Guide to Infection Prevention for Outpatient Settings: Minimum Expectations for Safe Care. Available at: *www.cdc.gov/HAI/settings/ outpatient/outpatient-care- guidelines.html*

Centers for Disease Control and Prevention. 2007 Guideline for Isolation Precautions: Preventing Transmission of Infectious Agents in Healthcare Settings. Available at: *www.cdc.gov/hicpac/pdf /isolation/Isolation2007.pdf*

Centers for Disease Control and Prevention. One and Only Injection Safety Campaign. Available at: *www.oneandonly campaign.org/*

(1) False; (2) False; (3) Never; (4) Always; (5) Never; (6) Never

Notes

Single-Use (Disposable) Devices

Examining the Issues

Single-use devices — also called disposable devices — offer great infection-control advantages over reusable clinical products. Because these items are used on only one patient and then discarded, they help to reduce the potential for patient-to-patient contamination. Examples of available single-use/disposable items for dentistry include syringe needles, face masks, prophy cups and brushes, plastic orthodontic brackets, and patient exam and surgical gloves.

Single-use devices typically are not heat-tolerant. They may be made of plastic or less expensive metals, they may be difficult to clean, and they generally are not designed to withstand between-patient processing (cleaning, disinfection/sterilization).

○ Never process (clean, disinfect/sterilize) and reuse single-use devices on another patient.

Needles are single-use items. To reduce the risk of injury, dispose of contaminated single-use sharps (including disposable burs) in the sharps container nearest the point of use.

To lower the risk of disease transmission, disposable devices for oral surgical procedures must be sterile at the time of use. Many of these disposable surgical devices are supplied sterile by the manufacturer.

Terms You Should Know

Cleaning

Contaminated

Disinfection

Disposable

Food and Drug Administration

Medical waste

Processing

Sharps

Single-use

Sterilization

For definitions, see "Glossary," beginning on page 166

The Bottom Line

Use single-use devices for one patient only and dispose of them appropriately.

Single-Use Items in Dentistry

These items are **ALWAYS** single-use/disposable in dentistry:

- Syringe needles
- Prophy cups and brushes
- Plastic orthodontic brackets
- Exam and surgical gloves
- Face masks
- Surface barriers
- Patient napkins
- Sharps containers (dispose of when fill-to line is reached; NEVER empty and reuse)
- Specimen containers
- Sterilization pouches
- Suture needles
- Irrigating syringes

These items are available in **EITHER DISPOSABLE OR REUSABLE** varieties:

- Air-water syringe tips
- High-volume evacuator tips
- Fluoride gel trays
- Impression trays
- Mirrors
- Prophy angles
- Saliva ejector tips
- Burs/diamonds
- Vacuum line traps

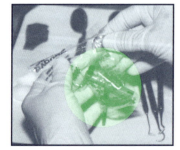

Disposable supplies like this prophy angle score high infection control points. They are used on only one patient and then discarded.

Disposables in Dental Settings

Advantages	Disadvantages
❏ **Prevents transfer of microorganisms from one patient to another via the device**	❏ **Possibly less efficient operation from a disposable device than from a reusable version**
❏ **Saves time; less processing**	❏ **Increased supply cost**
❏ **Most can be disposed of in the regular office trash***	❏ **More office waste**
* Consult your state and local regulations for advice on proper waste management in your area.	

Practice Tip

When an item is difficult to clean, consider switching to a disposable version.

Disposable tips for (a) saliva ejectors, (b) high-volume evacuators, and (c) air-water syringes are more efficient and effective dental infection control options.

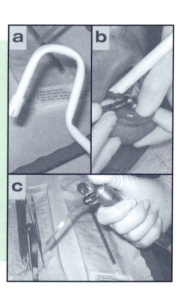

Common Questions and Answers

How do I dispose of contaminated single-use items?

In most areas, contaminated disposable items that are not sharps and are not soaked or caked with blood may be discarded with the regular office trash; there is no need to discard these items in a medical or biohazard container.

State and local regulations regarding medical waste — a term that refers to all waste generated in the diagnosis, treatment, or immunization of humans or animals — can vary. To ensure compliance, always consult the regulatory agency for your area.

For more information on managing waste in the dental practice setting, see Ch. 8, Environmental Infection Control.

Exercises in Understanding

1. Walk through your dental operatory. How many single-use/disposable items can you find? (Hint: Don't forget about PPE!)

2. In your practice setting, are the following devices reusable or single-use/disposable?

Air-water syringe tips	❑ Disposable	❑ Reusable
High-volume evacuator tips	❑ Disposable	❑ Reusable
Fluoride gel trays	❑ Disposable	❑ Reusable
Impression trays	❑ Disposable	❑ Reusable
Prophy angles	❑ Disposable	❑ Reusable

3. What advantages to single-use disposable items do you see in your average workday? What disadvantages? Talk to your Infection Control Coordinator about your observations.

Single-Use Disposables and My Work Day

My job title: _____

Advantages	Disdvantages
1.	1.
2.	2.
3.	3.
4.	4.
5.	5.
6.	6.

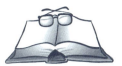

Recommended Readings and Resources

U.S. Department of Health and Human Services, Food and Drug Administration. Labeling recommendations for single-use devices reprocessed by third parties and hospitals; final guidance for industry and FDA, July 30, 2001.

Self-Test

Before moving on, test yourself with some questions on the material.
(answers appear below)

1. True or False: Disposables are an especially good infection control choice for items that are difficult to clean.

2. True or False: In most areas, contaminated disposable items that are caked or soaked with blood can be discarded with the regular office trash.

3. Which of the following is not a single-use/disposable item?

   a. patient exam gloves   b. bib   c. patient safety glasses   d. surface barrier

4. True or False: I can reuse a single-use/disposable item on a second patient if I clean it carefully and heat-sterilize it.

(1) True; (2) False; (3) c; (4) False.

Notes

Chapter 14

Preprocedural Mouthrinses

 ### Examining the Issues

Mouthrinses are used in dentistry for a number of reasons: to freshen breath, to prevent or control tooth decay, to reduce plaque formation on teeth and gums, to prevent or reduce gingivitis, or to deliver a combination of these effects. They also may promote infection control in the dental operatory.

Some mouthrinses — those containing an antimicrobial agent — have antiseptic properties that help reduce the number of microorganisms on the surface of oral tissues.

The use of preprocedural mouthrinses that reduce bacterial counts in the mouth also reduce the number of microorganisms that are released through aerosols, spatter, or direct contact. Preprocedural rinsing also may decrease the number of microorganisms introduced in the patient's bloodstream during invasive dental procedures.

Clinical research has not proven that use of a preprocedural mouthrinse prevents or reduces disease transmission from patients to staff. As such, CDC currently makes no recommendation for or against their routine use in dental practice.

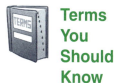 ### Terms You Should Know

Antimicrobial agent

Antiseptic

Bacterial endocarditis

Invasive procedure

Mouthrinse

Mucous membranes

Substantivity

Unit-dose

For definitions, see "Glossary," beginning on p. 166

 ### The Bottom Line

Dental practices may elect to routinely use preprocedural antimicrobial mouthrinses.

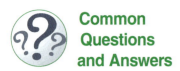

Common Questions and Answers

Can we use an "over-the-counter" drugstore mouthwash for a preprocedural rinse?

Some are suitable, others are not. Although over-the-counter mouthrinses that carry antiseptic claims contain agents that are effective in reducing bacterial counts, in many the effect may not last the duration of some lengthy dental procedures.

These rinses may be suitable for shorter, less involved patient appointments (for example, exams, appliance fitting, orthodontic adjustments). If opting to use an antimicrobial mouthrinse prior to oral surgical procedures, however, use a formula with greater substantivity, such as those containing chlorhexidine gluconate, essential oils, or povidone-iodine.

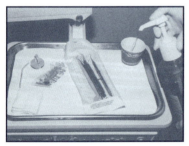

Adding a preprocedural mouthrinse to your operatory set-up can reduce the number of microorganisms in the patient's mouth, thus limiting the amount that can contaminate the environment or enter the patient's bloodstream.

Preprocedural Mouthrinses: What, when, where, why, and how

WHAT	A mouthrinse with antiseptic properties and residual activity. Currently, these agents include: ○ Chlorhexidine gluconate ○ Essential oils ○ Povidone-iodine
WHEN	Before any dental procedure, but preprocedural mouthrinsing may be most beneficial when rubber dam cannot be used and high-volume evacuation is not commonly employed. For example, before prophylaxis with a prophy cup or ultrasonic scaler.
WHERE	In the operatory, after seating the patient and before beginning examination and treatment.
WHY	To reduce the number of microorganisms in the patient's mouth, which in turn, reduces the number of organisms released through aerosols, droplet spatter, and direct contact. Reducing the number of microorganisms in the mouth may also reduce the number of microorganisms that are released into the patient's bloodstream when breaks in the mucous membrane occur during treatment.
HOW	Unit-dosed in a disposable cup.

Mouthrinse Precautions

○ **Alcohol in mouthrinses has limited antibacterial activity**. Although alcohol is found in most mouthrinses, it is merely a vehicle. Look for another antimicrobial agent (such as chlorhexidine gluconate, povidone-iodine, or essential oils) in preprocedural mouthrinse formulations. These agents have been shown to reduce the number of microorganisms in the mouth.

○ **Many over-the-counter "cosmetic mouthrinses" are not ideal preprocedural mouthrinses**. Formulated to mask oral malodor ("bad breath"), these mouthwashes have a pleasant taste and scent. Some carry antimicrobial claims, and while they may reduce bacterial counts, their substantivity is lower than that of other categories of mouthrinses.

○ **Although they can dramatically reduce tooth decay in both children and adults, fluoride mouthrinses have little to no antimicrobial activity**. Fluoride mouthrinses are not a suitable choice for a preprocedural mouthrinse aimed at reducing oral bacterial counts.

○ **Never give a preprocedural mouthrinse containing alcohol to patients when alcohol-containing products are contraindicated** (for example, salivary gland dysfunction, recovering alcoholics). Instead, look for an alcohol-free mouthrinse that contains antiseptic agents.

Exercises in Understanding

If a preprocedural mouthrinse is used in your practice setting:

1. Take a look at the label.

   What is the active ingredient? _____

   Does the active ingredient have antibacterial properties?   ❑ Yes   ❑ No

   Does the mouthrinse contain alcohol?   ❑ Yes   ❑ No

2. How does your practice setting make sure it doesn't give an alcohol-containing mouthrinse when it is contraindicated?

   _____

Self-Test

Before moving on, test yourself with some questions on the material.
(answers appear below)

1. True or False: Fluoride mouthrinses are suitable preprocedural mouthrinses.

2. In preprocedural mouthrinses, which of the following ingredients does not offer appropriate antibacterial properties?
   a. alcohol   c. povidone-iodine
   b. chlorhexidine gluconate   d. essential oils

3. Provide a preprocedural mouthrinse to patients in a _____ cup.
   a. glass   b. reusable   c. disposable   d. sterilizable

4. Ingredients that inhibit the growth of bacteria even after they are rinsed away are said to have:

   a. transient activity   c. tuberculocidal activity
   b. turbidity   d. substantivity

(1) False; (2) a; (3) c; (4) d.

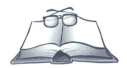

Recommended Readings and Resources

Fine DH, Furgang D, Korik I, Olshan A, Barnett ML, Vincent JW. Reduction of viable bacteria in dental aerosols by preprocedural rinsing with an antiseptic mouthrinse. *Am J Dent* 1993;6:219.

Fine DH, Yip J, Furgang D, Barnett ML, Olshan AM, Vincent J. Reducing bacteria in dental aerosols: pre-procedural use of an antiseptic mouth rinse. *JADA* 1993;124:56.

Litsky BY, Mascis JD, Litsky W. Use of an antimicrobial mouthwash to minimize the bacterial aerosol contamination generated by the high-speed drill. *Oral Surg Oral Med Oral Pathol* 1970;29:25.

Logothetis DD, Martinez-Welles JM. Reducing bacterial aerosol contamination with a chlorhexidine gluconate pre-rinse. *JADA* 1995;126:1634.

Klyn SL, Cummings DE, Richardson BW, Davis RD. Reduction of bacteria-containing spray produced during ultrasonic scaling. *Gen Dent* 2001;49:648.

Lockhart PB. An analysis of bacteremias during dental extractions. A double-blind, placebo-controlled study of chlorhexidine. *Arch Intern Med* 1996;156:513-20.

Wilson W, Taubert KA, Gewitz, M, Lockhart PB et al. Prevention of infective endocarditis: guidelines from the American Heart Association. *Circulation. 2007 Oct 9;116(15):1736-54.*

Notes

Chapter 15

Oral Surgical Procedures

 ## Examining the Issues

The oral cavity is colonized with numerous microorganisms. Oral surgical procedures involve the incision, excision, or reflection of tissue that exposes the areas of the oral cavity that normally are not exposed.

Examples of oral surgical procedures include:
- biopsy;
- periodontal surgery;
- apical surgery;
- implant surgery; and
- surgical tooth extractions (for example, removing an erupted or nonerupted tooth by elevating the mucoperiosteal flap, removing bone or a section of tooth, and suturing if needed).

By opening tissues that normally are not exposed, oral surgical procedures create an opportunity for microorganisms — both foreign organisms as well as those that typically exist in the mouth — to enter the patient's bloodstream, bone, and other tissue. This increases the potential for local or systemic infection.

Because of the increased potential for infection, stricter hand hygiene measures, sterile surgical gloves, and the use of sterile coolant/irrigating solution are warranted.

When performing oral surgical procedures:
- Perform surgical hand antisepsis using an antimicrobial product.
  - Use an antimicrobial soap and water,
    — or —
  - Use plain soap and water followed by an alcohol-based hand scrub with persistent activity.

- Wear sterile surgeon's gloves (see Ch. 5, Personal Protective Equipment, for review).

- Use sterile saline or sterile water as a coolant/irrigator.

- Use devices specifically designed to deliver sterile irrigating fluids. Remember: Because of biofilm contamination, there is no way to deliver sterile water via standard dental unit waterlines (See Ch. 9, Dental Unit Waterlines, Biofilm, and Water Quality, for a detailed explanation.) To deliver sterile coolant/irrigating fluids to surgical patients, use:
  - a sterile bulb syringe or irrigating syringe,
  - single-use disposable products, and/or
  - a sterile water delivery system (with disposable or sterilizable tubing).

In addition, to reduce the risk of post-surgical infection associated with implant placement, spore test with every sterilizer load that contains an implantable device, and avoid placing the device until after results of the spore test are known.

 ## The Bottom Line

Because of the potential added risk of infection from cutting or otherwise penetrating tissues that are not normally exposed, a higher level of precautions must be implemented to ensure patient protection.

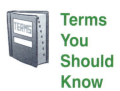 ## Terms You Should Know

Antiseptic handwash

Local

Oral surgical procedure

Reflection

Sterile water delivery system

Sterile surgical gloves

Surgical hand scrub

Systemic

For definitions, see "Glossary," beginning on page 166

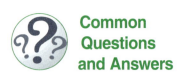

Common Questions and Answers

If I assist on an oral surgical procedure, must I also wear sterile surgical gloves and perform surgical hand antisepsis?

Yes. Any dental worker who will have his or her hands in the patient's mouth or will touch items used in the oral cavity during an oral surgical procedure must wear sterile surgeon's gloves and perform surgical hand antisepsis before gloving.

Although you must use an antimicrobial product, it is up to the worker/facility to choose whether to handwash using an antimicrobial soap and water or to wash hands with plain soap and water, then apply an alcohol-based hand rub before putting on new sterile gloves.

To further reduce the risk of post-surgical infection, sterile irrigating fluids should be used during all oral surgical procedures.

Step by Step

Surgical Hand Antisepsis: Hand Rub Technique

Before performing surgical procedures:

1 Remove rings, watches, and bracelets.

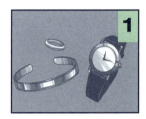

2 Remove debris from under fingernails using a nail cleaner under running water.

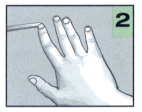

3 Perform surgical hand antisepsis using either an antimicrobial soap or an alcohol-based hand rub with persistent activity.

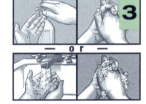

When using an antimicrobial soap:

Scrub hands, wrists, and forearms for time recommended by the manufacturer (usually 2-6 min.).
○ **NOTE**: Long scrub times (e.g., 10 min.) are not necessary.

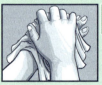

Dry thoroughly with sterile towels before donning sterile gloves.

When using an alcohol-based surgical hand rub:

4 Follow the manufacturer's instructions.

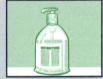

5 Before applying the alcohol solution, prewash hands and forearms with plain soap and water, then dry hands and forearms completely.

6 After applying the alcohol-based product as recommended, allow hands and forearms to dry thoroughly before putting on sterile surgical gloves.

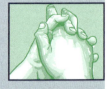

Infection Control Precautions:
Surgical vs. Nonsurgical Dental Procedures

SURGICAL DENTAL PROCEDURES	NONSURGICAL DENTAL PROCEDURES
BEFORE	
Perform surgical hand antisepsis: ○ Wash hands, wrists, and exposed areas of the forearms to the elbows using water and an antimicrobial handwashing agent such as chlorhexidine, iodine and iodophors, chloroxylenol [PCMX], or triclosan for 2 to 6 min. — or — ○ Wash hands using water and plain soap (non-antimicrobial) followed by an alcohol-based hand rub with persistent activity. Follow manufacturer instructions for the amount and duration of the hand rub	**If hands are not visibly soiled:** ○ Wash hands with soap (plain or antimicrobial) and water — or — ○ Use an alcohol-based hand rub. **If hands are visibly dirty, contaminated, or soiled** with blood or other body fluids: ○ Wash hands with either a non-antimicrobial soap and water or an antimicrobial soap and water.
Put on a new pair of sterile surgical gloves for each patient	**Put on a new pair of non-surgical examination gloves** for each patient
DURING	
Use devices specifically designed to deliver sterile irrigating fluids to the operating field. For example: ○ a bulb syringe or sterile irrigating syringe, ○ single-use disposable products, and/or ○ a sterile water delivery system (with disposable or sterilizable tubing)	**Use water from a dental unit that is regularly maintained and monitored** to deliver water that is of comparable or better microbiological quality than drinking water (500 CFU/mL or less)
If gloves become torn, punctured, or otherwise compromised during use: 1. Remove gloves immediately or as soon as feasible 2. Perform hand hygiene for surgical procedures 3. Put on a new pair of sterile surgical gloves before resuming treatment	**If gloves become torn, punctured, or otherwise compromised during use:** 1. Remove gloves immediately or as soon as feasible 2. Perform hand hygiene for non-surgical procedures (see p. 24 and 25) 3. Put on a new pair of exam gloves before resuming treatment

Delivering Sterile Solutions

Remember: Because of biofilm contamination, there is no way to deliver sterile water via standard dental unit waterlines. Use a bulb syringe or a sterile water delivery system to deliver coolant during oral surgical procedures.

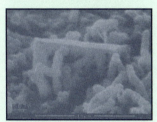

Microorganisms colonize the inside surface of the dental waterline, contaminating any sterile water that flows through it.

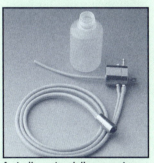

A sterile water delivery system, with a sterilizable water reservoir and autoclavable or disposable tubing is one way to ensure only sterile water reaches the surgical field.

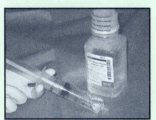

A sterile irrigating syringe can be used to draw sterile water from its reservoir and deliver it to the operating field during oral surgical procedures.

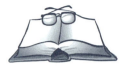

Recommended Readings and Resources

Centers for Disease Control and Prevention. Guideline for hand hygiene in health-care settings: Recommendations of the Health-care Infection Control Practices Advisory Committee and the HICPAC/SHEA/APIC/IDSA Hand Hygiene Task Force. *MMWR Morbid Mortal Weekly Rep* 2002;51 (No. RR-16).

Mangram AJ, Horan TC, Pearson ML, Silver LC, Jarvis WR. Guideline for prevention of surgical site infection, 1999. Hospital Infection Control Practices Advisory Committee. *Infect Control Hosp Epidemiol* 1999;20:250.

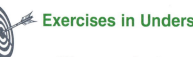

Exercises in Understanding

1. What types of oral surgical procedures are routinely performed in your practice?

_____

_____

_____

2. What method of hand hygiene is performed before oral surgical procedures in your practice? What products are used, what are their active ingredients (check the label), and for how long?

Hand Hygiene Action	Brand Name and Active Ingredient	Amount and Duration of Use
Antimicrobial handwash or surgical handscrub		
Alcohol hand rub preceded by soap and water handwash		

3. If your facility handles oral surgical cases, what are your sources of sterile water? How is it delivered to patients?

Self-Test

Before moving on, test yourself with some questions on the material.
(answers appear below)

1. Which of the following is not considered an oral surgical procedure?
   a. bone augmentation   b. implant placement   c. scaling   d. biopsy

2. Describe your hand hygiene choices before performing or assisting on an oral surgical procedure.

_____

_____

3. Why is it unadvisable to use sterile water delivered via the dental unit as coolant or irrigating solution during an oral surgical procedure?

_____

_____

4. For oral surgical procedures, always wear _____ gloves.
   a. non-sterile exam   b. sterile surgical   c. utility   d. any available

(1) c: (2) Surgical scrub technique using an antimicrobial handwash OR soap and water handwash followed by an alcohol-based hand rub used according to the manufacturer's instructions; (3) Microorganisms colonize the inside surface of the dental waterline, contaminating any sterile water that flows through it; (4) b.

Chapter 16

Handling of Biopsy Specimens

Examining the Issues

Dental infection control and safety sometimes extends beyond the walls of the practice setting. As a dental worker, your responsibility includes protecting those who transport, handle, and otherwise come into contact with infectious hazards generated through dental examination, diagnosis, and treatment.

Biopsy specimens are human tissue and therefore are potentially infectious. In the practice setting, handle them using proper infection control precautions.

❍ Always wear gloves when working with biopsy specimens.

When packaging specimens for transport to the laboratory, be sure they are securely contained to protect the persons who handle and transport them.

❍ Always use sturdy, leakproof, puncture-resistant containers with secure lids to keep specimens — and the hazards they present — contained during transport.

❍ Place the biohazard symbol on the container or on a bag that holds the container to identify the contents as infectious. This lets couriers, receivers, and laboratory personnel know that they must take proper precautions before opening and handling the materials inside.

❍ If the outside of the specimen container becomes contaminated, clean and disinfect the outside, or place it in a leakproof bag labeled with the biohazard symbol.

The Bottom Line

Dental workers must take responsibility for protecting those who handle, transport, or otherwise come into contact with infectious materials generated within the practice setting. This includes careful packaging and identification of contents as an infectious hazard.

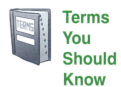

Terms You Should Know

Biohazard

Biohazard symbol

Biopsy

Specimen

For definitions, see "Glossary," beginning on page 166

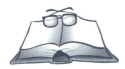

Recommended Readings and Resources

Occupational Safety and Health Administration 29 CFR Part 1910.1030 Occupational exposure to bloodborne pathogens; needlestick and other sharps injuries; final rule. *Federal Register* 2001; 66 (12); 5317-25 and *Federal Register* 1991 29 CFR Part 1910.1030 Occupational exposure to bloodborne pathogens; final rule. 56(235);64174-82. Available at *www.osha. gov/pls/oshaweb/owadisp.sho w_document?p_table=STA NDARDS&p_id=10051.*

Occupational Safety and Health Administration. Enforcement procedures for the Occupational Exposure to Bloodborne Pathogens CPL 2–2.69; November 27, 2001.

Infection Control Precautions

Preparing Specimens for Transport

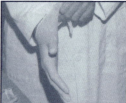

○ Always wear gloves when working with biopsy specimens.

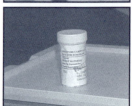

○ For transport to the lab, place biopsy specimens in a sturdy, leak-proof container labeled with the biohazard symbol.

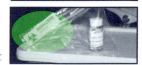

○ If the biopsy specimen container is visibly contaminated, place it in a leak-proof bag labeled with the biohazard symbol or clean and disinfect the outside of the container with a low- to intermediate-level disinfectant (see Ch. 8, Environmental Infection Control).

or

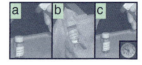

Exercises in Understanding

1. Where are leakproof specimen containers kept in your practice setting?

   _____

2. How does your practice identify infectious materials that are sent off-site? With biohazard bags, stickers, labels, or other?

   _____

Self-Test

Before moving on, test yourself with some questions on the material.
(answers appear below)

1. Biopsy specimen containers should be:
   a. reusable   b. child-proof   c. leakproof   d. clear

2. If the outside of a specimen container becomes contaminated:
   a. soak it in glutaraldehyde
   b. clean and then disinfect the outside surface using a low-
      to intermediate-level disinfectant
   c. immediately throw it away
   d. any of the above

3. True or False: A specimen container that has been contaminated on its outside surface may be placed in another bag, labeled with the biohazard symbol, and sent to the lab by the usual means.

(1) c; (2) b; (3) True.

Chapter 17

Handling of Extracted Teeth

Examining the Issues

Extracted teeth are regulated medical waste in the dental office. Regulated waste requires special storage, handling, neutralization, and disposal as covered by federal, state, and local rules and regulations on medical waste management and disposal (see Ch. 8, Environmental Infection Control).

Because they are a potentially infectious material, extracted teeth must be disposed of in medical waste containers.

Extracted teeth may be returned to your patient upon request. Once the teeth are given to the patient, waste management regulations for the dental office no longer apply.

Extracted teeth sometimes are sent to a dental laboratory for shade or size comparisons. These teeth should be cleaned, surface disinfected with an Environmental Protection Agency (EPA)-registered hospital disinfectant with intermediate-level activity (i.e., a tuberculocidal claim), and then packaged for transport to the dental laboratory.

Never place extracted teeth containing dental amalgam in a medical waste container that will be autoclaved or incinerated by the hauler/disposal service. High temperatures will release mercury vapors, which are a health hazard. Some commercial metal recycling companies may accept extracted teeth with metal restorations, including amalgam.
○ Check with your practice setting's metal recycler to see if the company will accept teeth containing metal fillings. Follow the hauler's instructions for proper disposal procedures within the clinical setting.
○ Consult your state and local regulations on the disposal of the amalgam.

Extracted teeth are occasionally collected for use in preclinical training of dental workers. Teeth that do not contain amalgam are preferred for educational purposes because they can be safely autoclaved. Step-by-step instructions for preparing extracted teeth for use in educational settings are detailed on the following pages.

Terms You Should Know

Biohazard symbol

Environmental Protection Agency (EPA)

Hospital disinfectant

Intermediate-level disinfectant

Mercury

Regulated medical waste

Tuberculocidal

For definitions, see "Glossary," beginning on page 166

The Bottom Line

Extracted teeth are considered infectious and are classified as regulated medical waste. Always follow state and local regulations for proper disposal, and maintain records of all medical waste transports for disposal (see Ch. 8, "Environmental Infection Control"). While special procedures are required to render extracted teeth non-infectious for reuse in dental educational settings, teeth containing amalgam must never be autoclaved.

At a Glance

Handling Extracted Teeth

○ **Dispose of extracted teeth as regulated medical waste** unless returned to the patient.

○ **Do not dispose of extracted teeth containing amalgam in regulated medical waste container intended for incineration**.

○ **When sending extracted teeth to a dental school or laboratory, clean and place the teeth in a leakproof container labeled with a biohazard symbol** and containing an appropriate disinfectant.

○ **Heat sterilize teeth that do not contain amalgam** before they are used for educational purposes.

○ **Never heat sterilize extracted teeth that contain amalgam** fillings.

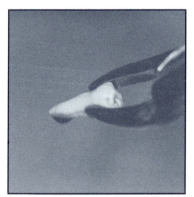

As human tissue, extracted teeth are considered infectious and are classified as regulated medical waste.

Step by Step

Preparing and Using Extracted Teeth in Educational Settings

For teeth that <u>do not contain</u> amalgam restorations:

1 Clean extracted teeth until they are free of visible blood and gross debris, then keep them moist in a closed container.

2 Place extracted teeth in a well-constructed container with a secure lid to prevent leaking during transport. Label the container with the biohazard symbol.

3 Before being used in an educational setting, heat-sterilize the teeth using an autoclave cycle for 40 min. This discourages microbial growth without compromising the tooth's physical properties.

4 When using the teeth in preclinical exercises, students should apply standard precautions, even though the extracted teeth have been made safe for handling. Applying standard precautions will more accurately simulate the clinical experience.

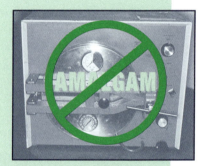

Never heat sterilize teeth containing amalgam. Mercury vaporization and exposure is a health hazard. For similar reasons, do not dispose of teeth containing amalgam in medical waste containers that the disposal service will incinerate.

For teeth that <u>contain amalgam</u> restorations:

1 Consult the manufacturer-supplied Material Safety Data Sheet on formalin for information on hazards, precautions, and disposal.

2 Immerse extracted teeth containing amalgam in 10% formalin solution for 2 weeks (14 days) to disinfect both the internal and external structures.

○ Formalin is the only liquid germicide shown to be effective in disinfecting both the interior and exterior of extracted teeth with amalgam, making them safe for use in educational settings. Liquid chemical germicides such as glutaraldehyde and diluted bleach (sodium hypochlorite) only disinfect the exteriors of extracted teeth, not the interior pulp tissue.

3 When using the teeth in preclinical exercises, students should apply standard precautions, even though the extracted teeth have been made safe for handling. Applying standard precautions will more accurately simulate the clinical experience.

Common Questions and Answers

Can I dispose of extracted teeth in our facility's sharps containers?

If your medical waste handler uses heat to sterilize the contents, teeth with amalgam fillings cannot be disposed of in the sharps container.

The commercial metal recycler your facility contracts with to remove scrap metals may be able to assist with disposal of amalgam-containing teeth. Along with scrap amalgam and other metals used in the dental setting, some (but not all) metal recyclers accept extracted teeth containing amalgam. While your recycler may be equipped to manage the toxicity of scrap metals, it is still the dental worker's responsibility to eliminate the infectious hazard. Always confirm with your recycler that the company accepts extracted teeth with amalgam restorations.

Exercises in Understanding

1. How are extracted teeth handled in your practice setting?

   Are they given to the patient?   ❑ Yes   ❑ No

   Are they donated to a dental school?   ❑ Yes   ❑ No

   Are they disposed of as regulated medical waste? ❑ Yes   ❑ No

2. When extracted teeth are sent to the dental lab for shade or size matching, what disinfectant is used?

   _____

   What is its EPA registration number? (Hint: Check the disinfectant's label.)

   _____

   What is its contact time?

   _____

3. How are extracted teeth disposed of …

   … if they do not have amalgam fillings? _____

   _____

   … if they contain amalgam fillings? _____

   _____

Self-Test

Before moving on, test yourself with some questions on the material.
(answers appear below)

As demonstrated in question 1, draw a line to match the processing method with the intended purpose of extracted teeth.

1. Amalgam-containing teeth for teaching   No processing required
2. Amalgam-free teeth for teaching   10% formalin for 2 weeks
3. Teeth for dental lab shade/size matching   Heat sterilize for 40 min
4. Teeth given to the patient   Intermediate-level disinfection

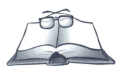

Recommended Readings and Resources

American Dental Association. Best Management Practices for Amalgam Waste (October 2007). Available at: *www.ada.org/~/media/ADA/ Member%20Center/FIles/topics_amalgamwaste_ brochure.ashx*

Cuny E, Carpenter WM. Extracted teeth: decontamination, disposal and use. *J Calif Dent Assoc* 1997;25:801.

Dominici JT, Eleazer PD, Clark SJ, Staat RH, Scheetz JP. Disinfection/ sterilization of extracted teeth for dental student use. *J Dent Educ* 2001;65:1278.

Pantera EA Jr, Schuster GS. Sterilization of extracted human teeth. *J Dent Educ* 1990;54:283.

Schulein TM. Infection control for extracted teeth in the teaching laboratory. *J Dent Educ* 1994;58:411.

Tate WH, White RR. Disinfection of human teeth for educational purposes. *J Dent Educ* 1991;55:583.

Healthcare Environmental Resource Center. Dental Offices – Regulated Medical Waste. Available at: *www.hercenter.org/ dental/index.cfm*

(1) 10% formalin for 2 weeks; (2) Heat sterilize for 40 min.; (3) Intermediate-level disinfection; (4) No processing required.

Notes

Chapter 18

Dental Laboratory

Examining the Issues

From dental office to dental lab and back, improper handling of contaminated impressions, prostheses, or appliances offers an opportunity for transmission of microorganisms.

Oral microorganisms have been found on and in dental impressions. These organisms can be transferred to dental casts, where some microbes can live within the gypsum for up to 7 days. Dental prostheses or impressions brought into the laboratory can be contaminated with bacteria, viruses, and fungi. Bringing untreated items into the laboratory increases the chances of cross-contamination.

Items sent to and returned from the dental lab — as well as any equipment used to process impressions, appliances, and prostheses — must be handled in a manner that prevents exposure of workers, patients, or the office environment to potential pathogens.

The Bottom Line

Effective communication and coordination between the laboratory and the clinical dental setting is the key to safe handling of materials that enter and leave the office or laboratory, and before patient use. Good communication ensures that the right cleaning and disinfection procedures are performed, that materials are not damaged or distorted during the disinfection process, and that effective disinfection procedures are not unnecessarily duplicated.

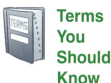

Terms You Should Know

Appliance

Bioburden

Cross-contamination

Hospital disinfectant

Impression

Personal protective equipment

Prosthesis

For definitions, see "Glossary," beginning on page 166

Shipping Dental Impressions

If clinical materials like dental impressions are not decontaminated before they are mailed, they are subject to federal regulations on the transport and shipping of infectious materials.

According to these regulations, containers for storage, transport, or shipping must be:

○ labeled with the biohazard symbol or color-coded red, and

○ closed prior to being stored, transported, or shipped.

If the outside of the primary container becomes contaminated, place the primary container inside a second container to prevent leaks during handling, processing, storage, transport, or shipping.

○ Label this second outside container or color-code it to identify the contents as a biohazard.

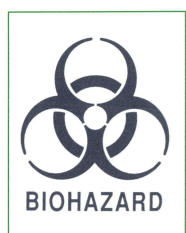

The universal biohazard symbol identifies items as infectious.

Precautions

To contain contamination in the dental setting...

Before handling cases in the in-office laboratory or sending them to an off-site laboratory:

○ **Thoroughly clean prostheses, impressions, orthodontic appliances, and other prosthodontic material**s (such as occlusal rims, temporary prostheses, bite registrations, and extracted teeth) to remove blood and bioburden.

○ **After cleaning, disinfect them using an EPA-registered intermediate-level hospital disinfectant** according to the manufacturer's instructions.

○ **Thoroughly rinse the items** to remove residual disinfectant.

   NOTE: Impression material/disinfectant compatibility can vary greatly, so always follow the manufacturers' recommendations for proper disinfection.

○ **Inform the lab**, in writing, about the specific methods that have been used to clean and disinfect the impression, stone model, or appliance. Send this information along with the case.

○ **Determine which office is responsible for final disinfection** processes:
   ❏ If dental laboratory staff disinfects a case before returning it to the doctor, they should cite the Environmental Protection Agency (EPA)-registered hospital disinfectant used and place the case in a tamper-evident container for shipment to the dental office.
   ❏ If such documentation is not received from the lab, the dental office is responsible for final disinfection procedures.

○ **Heat-sterilize heat-tolerant items used in the mouth** (such as metal impression trays and face bow forks) before using them on another patient.

To contain contamination in the dental lab:

○ **Establish a dedicated receiving and disinfecting area** to reduce contamination in the production area.

○ **Clean and disinfect the case before handling**, unless the doctor's written directions state that it has already been done.

○ **If a previously undetected area of blood or bioburden becomes apparent on the material or appliance, repeat cleaning and disinfection** procedures.

○ **Between cases, heat-sterilize (preferred) or high-level disinfect laboratory items** such as burs, polishing points, rag wheels, laboratory knives that are used on contaminated or potentially contaminated appliances, prostheses, or other material. Disposable laboratory items also may be used.

○ **Disinfect heat-sensitive lab items** exposed to patient materials.

○ **Between cases, clean and disinfect pressure pots and water baths.** These items are particularly susceptible to contamination with microorganisms.
   ❐ Use an EPA-registered low-level hospital disinfectant labeled effective against HIV and HBV, or an EPA-registered intermediate-level (tuberculocidal claim) hospital disinfectant.

○ **Barrier-protect or clean and disinfect environmental surfaces** in the same manner as in the dental treatment area (see Ch. 8, Environmental Infection Control).

○ **Discard waste with the general office trash** unless waste generated in the dental laboratory (for example, disposable trays, impression material) falls under the category of regulated medical waste (see p. 70).

○ **Dispose of sharp items such as burs, disposable blades, and orthodontic wires in puncture-resistant containers.**

1

Step by Step

Processing Dental Impressions

To make dental impressions safe for handling:

1 Rinse the impression under running tap water to clean it. If you need to, use a soft, camel-hair brush to remove debris.

2 Disinfect the impression using an intermediate-level hospital disinfectant for the contact time recommended on the germicide's label.

3 After the manufacturer-recommended contact time has elapsed, thoroughly rinse the disinfected impression under tap water to remove any residual antimicrobial chemicals.

4 After a thorough rinse, gently shake the impression within the sink basin to remove adherent water with minimal spatter.

NOTE: Unless the germicide is specifically approved for reuse, never reuse disinfectants to disinfect dental impressions.

Always consult the impression material manufacturer on the stability of specific materials during disinfection.

Impression Materials and Disinfectant Choices

The chart below lists the various types of impression materials and the tuberculocidal disinfectants that generally can be used to disinfect them.

NOTE: Impression material/disinfectant compatibility can vary even within the same generic product categories, so always follow manufacturer recommendations for proper disinfection.

Impression Material	Disinfecting agent
Alginate	iodophors; dilute sodium hypochlorite solution
Polysulfide	iodophors; complex phenolics*; dilute sodium hypochlorite solution
Silicone	iodophors; complex phenolics*; dilute sodium hypochlorite solution
Polyether	iodophors**; complex phenolics**; dilute sodium hypochlorite solution
ZOE impression paste	iodophors
Reversible hydrocolloid	iodophors; dilute sodium hypochlorite solution
Compound	iodophors; dilute sodium hypochlorite solution

* Prepared according to the manufacturer's instructions.
** Use with caution. Consult manufacturer's recommendations.

Personal Protective Equipment in the Dental Lab

Whether in the office or the dental laboratory, personal protective equipment (PPE) must be worn when handling lab cases that have not been disinfected.

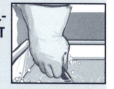
CHEMICAL-RESISTANT UTILITY GLOVES

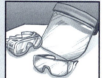
EYE / FACE PROTECTION

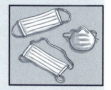
SURGICAL MASK

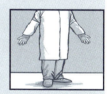
LAB COAT OR CLINIC JACKET

When to Disinfect

The best time to clean prostheses or appliances is as soon as possible after removal from the mouth, before blood or other bioburden can dry on the item's surface.

Always consult with manufacturers of impression materials regarding the stability of specific materials during disinfection.

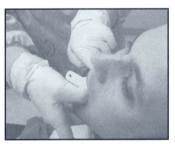

Disinfect impressions as soon as they are removed from the patient's mouth.

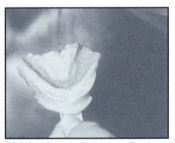

Disinfect impressions according to the material and germicide manufacturers' recommendations.

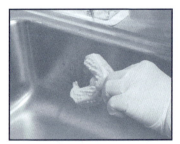

After the contact time has elapsed, rinse under tap water then gently shake to remove excess moisture.

Common Questions and Answers

Who should disinfect the final prosthesis before it is delivered to the patient? The dentist or the lab?

Either party can assume responsibility for disinfecting the final prosthesis. Talk to your dental laboratory to establish a protocol. Some practices find it makes sense for the dentist to disinfect impressions before they are sent to the lab and for the lab to disinfect the final prostheses before sending them back to the dentist.

Either way, both the dentist and the lab staff should document disinfection of any items transported between the two facilities. This helps eliminate duplication of efforts that could compromise impressions — and in turn, the final prostheses — without compromising patient or worker safety.

Should I disinfect impressions by spraying or immersing them in disinfectant?

Both immersion and spraying have been recommended for disinfection of impressions. To its advantage, spraying uses less solution, and often the same disinfectant can be used for general disinfection of operatory surfaces. Nonetheless, sprayed disinfectant tends to pool, which may prevent some surfaces (particularly in undercuts) from being adequately exposed to the germicide. In addition, spraying releases disinfectant into the air, which increases the chances for staff exposure to a hazardous chemical. As such, some organizations encourage immersion disinfection of all dental impressions.

A variety of containers can be used to disinfect impressions, although only well-sealed containers should be used for chemical baths. Glass beakers or plastic containers that can withstand contact with disinfectants can be used, processed, and reused to immerse impressions; alternatively, inexpensive, zipper-closure plastic bags provide an airtight, disposable option.

When using impression materials that may distort from immersion (such as polyethers), spraying may be the better alternative. The impression material manufacturer can offer suggestions on compatible disinfectants and disinfection techniques.

If spraying is recommended:
1. Spray the impression thoroughly and wrap it with well-moistened paper towels.
2. After the appropriate contact time, remove the impression and rinse it thoroughly with tap water. Shake gently to remove adherent water.
3. The impression is ready to be poured.

How long should I leave the disinfectant on the impression before rinsing?

Consult the disinfectant's label. Because hydrophilic materials such as polyether absorb water or disinfectant solution, disinfect these impressions using a product that requires no more than 10 min. contact time.

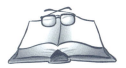

 ## Exercises in Understanding

1. What disinfectants are used to disinfect impressions in your practice setting?

   Type of impression material   Disinfectant name   Contact time

   1. _____

   2. _____

   3. _____

2. Do you disinfect cases before they are sent to the dental lab? If so, what documentation conveys this information to the laboratory worker who receives the case? (For example, do you attach a label or enclose a form? What does the form/label say?)

   _____

   _____

3. Are finished prostheses disinfected by the lab or in your practice setting? How do you know if the lab has disinfected the case?

   _____

   _____

 ## Self-Test

Before moving on, test yourself with some questions on the material.
(answers appear below)

1. Use personal protective equipment in the laboratory until _____.

2. Impressions should be disinfected with a(n) _____.

3. True or False: Impressions should be shipped to the lab with residual disinfectant still on their surfaces to make sure that any remaining microorganisms have been killed.

4. How often should labs disinfect pressure pots and water baths?

5. True or False: Just like a dental practice's instrument processing area, a dental lab should set up its receiving area to take items from "dirty" to "clean."

Recommended Readings and Resources

Fluent MT, Molinari JA. How the Dental laboratory Provides Infection Control. Inside Dental Assisting. 2013;9(2). Available at: *www.dentalaegis.com/ida/2013/04/how-the-dental-laboratory-provides-infection-control*

Kugel G, Perry RD, Ferrari M, Lalicata P. Disinfection and communication practices: a survey of U.S. dental laboratories. *JADA* 2000;131:786.

Merchant VA. Infection Control in the Dental Laboratory. In: Molinari JA. Practical Infection Control in Dentistry. 3rd ed. Philadelphia, PA: Lippincott, Williams and Wilkins; 2010:246-260.

Plummer KD, Wakefield CW. Practical infection control in dental laboratories. *Gen Dent* 1994;42:545.

Powell GL, Runnells RD, Saxon BA, Whisenant BK. The presence and identification of organisms transmitted to dental laboratories. *J Prosthet Dent* 1990; 64(2):235.

(1) all items to be handled have been disinfected; (2) EPA-registered, intermediate-level hospital disinfectant; (3) False; (4) Between cases; (5) True.

Notes

Chapter 19

Tuberculosis and Dentistry

Examining the Issues

Tuberculosis (TB) is a contagious disease caused by the *Mycobacterium tuberculosis* bacterium. The bacteria are carried in microscopic airborne particles called droplet nuclei. Through a productive cough, these droplet nuclei can be aerosolized from persons with TB of the lungs or larynx (voicebox) and can stay suspended in the air for several hours, where others can breathe them into their lungs. Some people may become very ill ("active tuberculosis"). In most people, however, the body's immune response usually prevents the bacteria from spreading outside the lungs to other parts of the body or to other persons. Even though the infected person isn't sick or contagious, the bacteria can remain alive in the lungs for many years ("latent tuberculosis infection"). Many people with latent TB infection never develop TB disease. In these people, the TB bacteria remain alive but inactive for a lifetime without causing disease. In others, however, especially those who have weak immune systems, the bacteria can become active and cause disease.

The test for TB is the tuberculin skin test (TST, described on page 127). A positive test could mean either active or latent TB infection; the test cannot recognize the difference between the contagious (active) and the noncontagious (latent) forms of TB. Symptoms of active TB include a productive cough, night sweats, fatigue, malaise, fever, and unexplained weight loss. While persons with latent TB infection will have a positive skin test, they have none of these symptoms and are not contagious. Although they cannot transmit the disease to others, persons with latent TB infection may still need to receive antibiotics to treat the infection. Without proper treatment, a latent infection may eventually develop into active (contagious) disease in some individuals.

TB risk in dentistry

Only one report of TB transmission from a dental worker to patients and one report of transmission between dental workers have ever been documented. Patients with active TB are typically too sick to seek elective dental care. Nonetheless, patients infected with TB may occasionally come to an outpatient dental facility for emergency dental treatment. Understanding the disease and recognizing its symptoms can help dental healthcare workers to make informed decisions about patient management. This is especially important because while standard precautions protect against body fluid exposures, they do not protect against airborne diseases like TB.

CDC recommends that dental practices have a written TB infection control plan.

The Bottom Line

Although the risk of TB transmission in dentistry is likely very low, your practice setting should routinely perform risk assessments to determine its TB infection control policies. Such policies cover how dental workers in your facility detect and refer patients who may have active tuberculosis, how they manage dental emergencies in patients with active tuberculosis, and dental worker TB education, training, counseling, and screening.

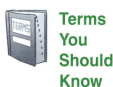

Terms You Should Know

Administrative controls

Droplet nuclei

Environmental controls

Malaise

N-95 respirator

Occupational risk

Personal respiratory protection

Tuberculosis

  Active

  Latent

For definitions, see "Glossary," beginning on page 166

Signs and Symptoms of TB

A person with active TB disease is contagious. Symptoms of active TB disease include:

○ a productive cough,

○ bloody sputum,

○ night sweats,

○ fatigue,

○ malaise,

○ fever,

○ unexplained weight loss.

Without these symptoms, in particular the productive cough, which expels the TB bacteria from the lungs and into the air, a TB patient is not considered contagious.

If urgent dental treatment is required for a patient who has, or is suspected of having active TB disease, refer the patient to a facility (such as a hospital) that is equipped for transmission-based precautions and can provide airborne infection isolation. This protocol includes:

○ TB isolation rooms, negatively pressured relative to the corridors, and air either exhausted to the outside or HEPA-filtered if recirculation is necessary, and

○ respiratory protection such as a fit-tested, disposable N-95 respirator for all workers who come in contact with the patient. An N-95 respirator meets minimum filtration performance criteria for respiratory protection in TB areas. It filters 95% of the TB particles from the air you breathe.

Precautions

Preventing TB transmission in the dental setting

TB transmission is prevented using administrative controls, environmental controls, and personal respiratory protection. Your practice setting should have policies in place to direct you in referring or otherwise managing patients suspected of having active tuberculosis. Policies should also address tuberculin skin testing and follow-up for dental team members in the unlikely event that they encounter a patient with active TB while on the job, as well as those workers who have symptoms consistent with active TB.

Patient management

For the respiratory health of the dental team and to ensure that patients who are seriously ill receive the care they need:

○ **Routinely ask all patients whether they have a history of TB disease or symptoms suggestive of TB**. Inquire when taking patients' initial medical histories and at periodic updates thereafter.

○ **Promptly refer for medical evaluation any patient with a medical history or symptoms that suggest undiagnosed, untreated active TB**. Such patients should not remain in the dental-care facility any longer than required to evaluate the dental condition and arrange a referral.
  ❏ While in the dental healthcare facility, any patient suspected of having active TB should be isolated as well as possible.
  ❏ Ask the patient to wear a surgical mask when not being evaluated.
  ❏ Instruct the patient to cover his or her mouth and nose when coughing or sneezing.

○ **Defer all elective dental treatment until a physician confirms that the patient does not have infectious TB.** If the patient is diagnosed as having active TB, elective dental treatment should be deferred until the patient is no longer infectious.

○ **If urgent dental care must be provided for a patient who has or is suspected of having active TB disease, provide care only in a previously identified facility that has TB isolation rooms and special air filtration** (for example, a hospital). Standard precautions do not protect against TB transmission, so added precautions are necessary.
  ❏ Standard surgical face masks do not prevent TB transmission.
  ❏ Only fit-tested, disposable N-95 respirators or other appropriate respiratory protection guards against airborne disease agents.

Dental workers

For all dental workers with patient contact:

○ **Get a baseline two-step tuberculin skin test** at the beginning of employment. If an unprotected occupational exposure occurs, a positive result may then be distinguished from infection from a previous exposure.

For any dental worker who has a persistent cough for at least 3 weeks, especially in combination with other signs or symptoms consistent with active TB:

○ **Get evaluated immediately by a medical professional**.

○ **Do not return to the workplace** until either:
  ❏ a diagnosis of TB has been excluded, or
  ❏ medication has been initiated and a physician has indicated that the worker is not contagious.

Common Questions and Answers

How can I tell the difference between a patient with a cough from a cold and a patient with contagious TB?

Tuberculosis is a serious illness with a very deep, productive cough that often produces bloody sputum. The patient will experience much greater fatigue and malaise than with lesser respiratory illnesses, and likely will have lost significant weight. Also, with active TB, patients usually don't suffer the nasal congestion common with a head cold.

What if...

... I have been in contact with a patient I think has contagious TB? Will I get sick?

Verify with the patient's physician that the person actually has active tuberculosis. If so, you should be promptly evaluated by a medical professional and tested for infection.

If your tuberculin skin test is positive, you may be put on a course of medication to prevent active disease from developing. Because TB can be a very serious and contagious disease, you must strictly comply with all prescription medication orders, even if you don't feel sick. The antibiotic regimen your physician recommends is intended to keep you healthy and prevent latent infection from developing resistance to antibiotics.

Although TB is a contagious disease, it is not generally spread by casual contact. People with TB disease are most likely to spread it to family members, friends, coworkers, and other persons who they spend time with every day.

Exercises in Understanding

If a patient with active TB were to come to your practice setting, where would you perform your evaluation and have the patient wait? Remember: It's best to keep the patient away from other patients and dental workers.

_____

_____

Tuberculin Skin Test

The tuberculin skin test (TST) is used to identify or confirm infection in persons who have been exposed to or are suspected of having TB.

A small amount of purified liquid containing specific substances from the TB microorganism is injected between the layers of the skin of the forearm. A small welt forms almost immediately. In 48-72 hours, the results can be read. A positive TST reveals inflammation and a hardening of the skin of the affected area.

The TST identifies infection, but it can't discern between active (contagious) and latent (noncontagious) disease. Regardless of whether a patient feels sick, antibiotics may be prescribed to prevent latent infection from turning into active disease at a later date.

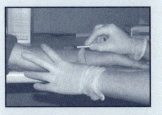

The TST is administered intradermally in the skin of the forearm.

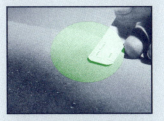

A patchy area of firm, fibrous tissue and inflammation indicates infection with TB.

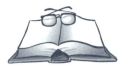

Recommended Readings and Resources

Centers for Disease Control and Prevention. Guidelines for preventing the transmission of *Mycobacterium tuberculosis* in health-care facilities, 1994. *MMWR Morbid Mortal Weekly Report* 1994;43 (No. RR-13). Available at: *www.cdc. gov/mmwr/preview/mmwrhtm l/00035909.htm.*

Centers for Disease Control and Prevention. Guidelines for Preventing the Transmission of Mycobacterium Tuberculosis in Health-Care Settings, 2005, available at: *www.cdc.gov/mmwr/pdf/rr/rr 5417.pdf*

Centers for Disease Control and Prevention. Basic TB Facts. Available at: *www.cdc.gov/tb/topic/ basics/default.htm*

Cleveland JL, Gooch BF, Bolyard EA, et al. TB infection control recommendations from the CDC, 1994: considerations for dentistry. *JADA* 1995;126:593.

Merte JL, Kroll CM, Collins AS, Melnick AL. An epidemiologic investigation of occupational transmission of Mycobacterium tuberculosis infection to dental health care personnel. *JADA 2014;145(5):464-471*

Smith WH, Davies D, Mason KD, Onions JP. Intraoral and pulmonary tuberculosis following dental treatment. *Lancet 1982;1:842-4.*

Self Test

1. Why is baseline tuberculin skin testing recommended for healthcare workers?

2. True or False: Persons with latent TB can transmit the disease.

3. If a patient suspected of having active TB arrives for a routine exam and prophylaxis:

   a. wear an N-95 respirator while treating the patient
   b. postpone the appointment and refer the patient for a medical evaluation
   c. refer the patient to the local hospital for the exam and cleaning
   d. contact the CDC

4. True or False: There has never been a case of TB transmission associated with dentistry.

5. The microscopic airborne particles that carry *Mycobacterium tuberculosis* out of the lungs and into the air are called:

   a. droplet nuclei   b. droplet spatter   c. bacilli   d. tuberculin

(1) In case of an exposure, knowing baseline test results could discern between an existing infection and a recent disease; (2) False; (3) b; (4) False; (5) a.

Chapter 20

Program Evaluation and Staff Training

Examining the Issues

The goal of a dental infection control program is to provide a safe working environment that reduces the risk of healthcare-associated infections among patients and occupational exposures among DHCP. To make sure that infection control procedures are being carried out as they should be — and to make sure that they're working — the infection control program in your facility should be continually evaluated.

Effective program evaluation helps to improve procedures and ensure that they remain useful, practical, and relevant in day-to-day dentistry. It is an essential organizational practice.

Continually evaluating your practice setting's infection control program allows constant improvements in the infection control program and in dental practice protocols. Deficiencies or problems in applying infection control principles and procedures are identified, so factors contributing to the problems can be modified as needed.

Infection Prevention Education and Training

Education and training on the basic principles and practices of infection control are critical elements of a successful infection control program. All DHCP in your practice should receive training on safe practices that prevent the spread of infection and protect staff and patients from injury.

Your practice should:
- Provide job- or task-specific infection control education and training to all workers, employees from outside agencies, contractors or volunteers.
- Provide safety training (e.g., OSHA bloodborne pathogens training) aimed at staff and patient safety.
- Provide education and training annually, during staff orientation, and when new tasks or procedures are implemented.
- Maintain training records according to state and federal requirements.

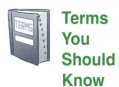

Terms You Should Know

Barrier

Engineering controls

Exposure control plan

Hand hygiene

Handwashing

Healthcare-associated infection

Immunization

Occupational exposure

Personal protective equipment

Postexposure management

Program evaluation

Safer medical devices

Sharps safety devices

Sterilization monitoring

Work practice controls

For definitions, see "Glossary," beginning on page 166

The Bottom Line

Regular evaluation of infection control protocols and procedures and staff training are important components of safe dentistry. Always cooperate with efforts to evaluate and improve infection control efforts in your practice setting.

Monitoring Infection Control in Practice

Your health and safety and the health and safety of the patients you treat should not be taken lightly. Use every workday to remain aware of the "hows" and "whys" of infection control in your dental setting, and bring any questions, concerns, and suggestions for improvements to your Infection Control Coordinator.

Some ways you can evaluate your facility's infection control program:

• Share your questions, observations, and ideas in staff meetings

• Watch for any signs of equipment or procedural problems and report these in the records you maintain

• Participate in the selection process for new devices.

CDC created a checklist to help you assess your dental setting and identify infection control lapses or deficient practices. You can view the checklist in Appendix B of this workbook, on the OSAP website or the CDC website.

Evaluating Your Infection Control Program

For a successful infection control program, your practice setting should be:

○ developing and applying standard operating procedures (such as using engineering and work practice controls);

○ evaluating practices as they are performed by staff;

○ documenting occupational exposures to blood and work-related illnesses in dental team members; and

○ monitoring healthcare-associated infections in patients.

To evaluate the infection control program in your practice setting, the dentist or Infection Control Coordinator may:

○ periodically observe infection control procedures as they are performed;

○ use checklists to document procedures; and

○ routinely review any occupational exposures to bloodborne pathogens to help reduce the risk of the future exposures.

Expectations for Safe Dental Care

Standard Precautions are recommended infection control practices for patient care, regardless of suspected or confirmed infection, anywhere health care is delivered. In the *Summary of Infection Prevention Practices in Dental Settings: Basic Expectations for Safe Care*, CDC offers a checklist to determine if your dental setting is meeting the minimum expectations for safe dental care. This checklist, also in Appendix B of this workbook, is designed to help you assess your dental setting and identify infection control lapses or deficient practices.
By using this checklist, you can

• Ensure that your dental setting has appropriate infection prevention policies and practices in place, including appropriate training and education of dental health care personnel (DHCP) on infection prevention practices.

• Ensure that your dental setting has adequate supplies to allow DHCP to provide safe care and a safe working environment. ⊠

• Systematically assess personnel compliance with the expected infection prevention practices and to provide feedback to DHCP regarding performance.

Lapses in Infection Control

Certain lapses infection control, such as reusing syringes on more than one patient, or failure to properly sterilize instruments can spread serious infections and should be corrected immediately. When lapses such as these are identified, immediately contact the state or local health department for consultation. Appropriate action must be taken to identify, notify and test potentially infected patients.

CDC has resources for evaluating and managing infection control breaches: www.cdc.gov/hai/outbreaks/steps_for_eval_ic_breach.html.

In addition, CDC has a Patient Notification Toolkit to assist with patient notification following identification of an infection control lapse or disease transmission: www.cdc.gov/injectionsafety/pntoolkit/index.html.

If lapses in infection control are identified in your dental setting:

- Determine risks posed to patients and staff

- Determine why the correct infection control practice was not being performed

- Demonstrate the correct practices

- Provide appropriate personnel training

Common Questions and Answers

Our infection control program is running smoothly. Why do we need to evaluate it?

Program evaluation is about applying checks and balances to existing practices and addressing new factors as they arise.

The dental product marketplace is constantly changing and growing; infection control products are no exception. As new devices, chemicals, and component materials are introduced, many can become part of your infection control program. New products — even those within the same general product category — can require changes in techniques, precautions, and associated work practices. Evaluating product performance as well as DHCP use of the new technology ensures that the products — and DHCP who use them — are performing to standard.

Similarly, new workers can join a dental team, sometimes introducing procedures from other practice settings that may not be part of your standard operating procedures. Observation and evaluation help to get everyone on the same page of the exposure control plan.

Some infection control procedures are so technique-sensitive that a simple lapse can cause the procedure to fail. Such is the case with use of parenteral medications and a number of currently available chemical protocols for waterline treatment, where failure to apply aseptic technique can result in serious contamination.

In other scenarios, time pressures can cause a DHCP to cut corners on infection control. Dentistry is fortunate in that it is a low-injury, low-risk profession. A major component of infection control training, however, is instilling the concept that "low risk does not equal no risk." Program evaluation provides the opportunity to reinforce good infection control and safety habits and correct any substandard ones, and that's an opportunity that should not be missed.

You've Done It!

Congratulations! You've completed *From Policy to Practice: OSAP's Guide to the Guidelines* and are now up to date on current recommendations from the Centers for Disease Control and Prevention, the United States' lead federal agency for protecting the health and safety of people.

Your hard work in studying and applying infection control principles in practice will pay off every day that you work in a dental setting. The information you have learned in this book also has prepared you to be a knowledgeable, aware patient when you yourself seek dental or medical care.

Thank you for using *From Policy to Practice: OSAP's Guide to the CDC Guidelines*. You can find a wealth of additional infection control educational materials, information, and training options at the OSAP website: *www.osap.org*.

Exercises in Understanding

1. List three ways that you, your team members, and your infection control manager continually evaluate the infection control program in your practice setting.

   (1) _____

   (2) _____

   (3) _____

2. Think about the last staff meeting at your practice setting. What infection control and safety issues were discussed? If problems or concerns were identified, how were they resolved?

   _____
   _____
   _____

3. What checklists are used or posted for infection control procedures?

   _____
   _____

Self Test

1. True or False: Staff meetings are not a good time to review procedures and discuss the facility's infection control program.

2. Name three reasons why infection control programs should be continually monitored, even if they appear to be working well.

   (1) _____

   (2) _____

   (3) _____

3. True or False: The practice setting's exposure control plan should be reviewed by staff for clarity.

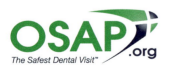

Creator and publisher of this workbook, OSAP is the nonprofit Organization for Safety and Asepsis Procedures. OSAP assumes no liability for actions taken based on information herein.

(1) False; (2) New, safer products may become available; new employees may join the staff; introducing procedures from other practice settings; some finer points of technique-sensitive procedures may need to be reviewed; frequent evaluation can remind dental health care personnel of the importance of infection control procedures and discourage shortcuts that could compromise patient and occupational health and safety; (3) True.

CDC Guidelines for Infection Control in Dental Health-Care Settings

The standard of practice for dental infection control is based upon recommendations published by CDC in the *Guidelines for Infection Control in Dental Health-Care Settings – 2003*. In 2016, CDC released the *Summary of Infection Prevention Practices in Dental Settings: Basic Expectations for Safe Care*. The summary covers basic infection control expectations for safe dental care as described in the *Guidelines for Infection Control in Dental Health-Care Settings – 2003* and includes relevant recommendations released by CDC since 2003. Although it includes some new recommendations, the summary should be considered a companion, not a replacement for the 2003 guideline document.

The following recommendations have been released by CDC since 2003:

Administrative Measures

1. Develop and maintain written infection prevention policies and procedures appropriate for the services provided by the facility and based upon evidence-based guidelines, regulations, or standards.

2. Infection prevention policies and procedures are re-assessed at least annually or according to state or federal requirements.

3. Assign at least one individual trained in infection prevention responsibility for coordinating the program.

4. Provide supplies necessary for adherence to Standard Precautions (e.g., hand hygiene products, safer devices to reduce percutaneous injuries, personal protective equipment).

5. Facility has system for early detection and management of potentially infectious persons at initial points of patient encounter.

Infection Prevention Education and Training

1. Maintain training records according to state and federal requirements.

Respiratory Hygiene/Cough Etiquette

1. Implement measures to contain respiratory secretions in patients and accompanying individuals who have signs and symptoms of a respiratory infection, beginning at point of entry to the facility and continuing throughout the visit.

2. Post signs at entrances with instructions to patients with symptoms of respiratory infection to:

    • Cover their mouths/noses when coughing or sneezing.

    • Use and dispose of tissues.

    • Perform hand hygiene after hands have been in contact with respiratory secretions.

3. Provide tissues and no-touch receptacles for disposal of tissues.

4. Provide resources for performing hand hygiene in or near waiting areas.

5. Offer masks to coughing patients and other symptomatic persons when they enter the dental setting.

6. Provide space and encourage persons with symptoms of respiratory infections to sit as far away from others as possible. If available, facilities may wish to place these patients in a separate area while waiting for care.

7. Educate DHCP on the importance of infection prevention measures to contain respiratory secretions to prevent the spread of respiratory pathogens when examining and caring for patients with signs and symptoms of a respiratory infection.

Safe Injection Practices

1. Prepare injections using aseptic technique in a clean area.

2. Disinfect the rubber septum on a medication vial with alcohol before piercing.

3. Do not reuse needles or syringes to enter a medication vial or solution, even when obtaining additional doses for the same patient.

4. Do not use single-dose (single-use) medication vials, ampules, and bags or bottles of intravenous solution for more than one patient.

5. Dedicate multidose vials to a single patient whenever possible.

6. If multidose vials will be used for more than one patient, they should be kept in a centralized medication area and should not enter the immediate patient treatment area to prevent inadvertent contamination

7. If a multidose vial enters the immediate patient treatment area it should be dedicated for single-patient use and discarded immediately after use.

8. Date multidose vials when first opened and discard within 28 days unless the manufacturer specifies a shorter or longer date for that opened vial.

Sterilization and Disinfection of Patient-Care Items and Devices

1. Have manufacturer instructions for reprocessing reusable dental instruments/equipment readily available, ideally in or near the reprocessing area.

2. Label sterilized items with the sterilizer used, the cycle or load number, the date of sterilization, and, if applicable, the expiration date.

3. Ensure routine maintenance for sterilization equipment is performed according to manufacturer instructions and maintenance records are available.

Guidelines for Infection Control in Dental Health-Care Settings - 2003

The following recommendations are excerpted from CDC's Guidelines for Infection Control in Dental Health-Care Settings—2003. MMWR 2003;52(No. RR-17):1–76. These evidence-based recommendations represent the standard of care for infection control in dental settings. For references and discussion of the science supporting each recommendation, see the original document, available at: www.cdc.gov/mmwr/PDF/ rr/rr5217.pdf.

Recommendations

Each recommendation is categorized on the basis of existing scientific data, theoretical rationale, and applicability. Rankings are based on the system used by CDC and the Healthcare Infection Control Practices Advisory Committee (HICPAC) to categorize recommendations:

Category IA. Strongly recommended for implementation and strongly supported by well-designed experimental, clinical, or epidemiologic studies.

Category IB. Strongly recommended for implementation and supported by experimental, clinical, or epidemiologic studies and a strong theoretical rationale.

Category IC. Required for implementation as mandated by federal or state regulation or standard. When IC is used, a second rating can be included to provide the basis of existing scientific data, theoretical rationale, and applicability. Because of state differences, the reader should not assume that the absence of a IC implies the absence of state regulations.

Category II. Suggested for implementation and supported by suggestive clinical or epidemiologic studies or a theoretical rationale.

Unresolved issue. No recommendation. Insufficient evidence or no consensus regarding efficacy exists.

I. Personnel Health Elements of an Infection-Control Program

A. General Recommendations

1. Develop a written health program for dental health-care personnel that includes policies, procedures, and guidelines for education and training; immunizations; exposure prevention and postexposure management; medical conditions, work-related illness, and associated work restrictions; contact dermatitis and latex hypersensitivity; and maintenance of records, data management, and confidentiality (IB).
2. Establish referral arrangements with qualified health-care professionals to ensure prompt and appropriate provision of preventive services, occupationally related medical services, and postexposure management with medical follow-up (IB, IC).

B Education and Training

1. Provide dental health-care personnel 1) on initial employment, 2) when new tasks or procedures affect the employee's occupational exposure, and 3) at a minimum, annually, with education and training regarding occupational exposure to potentially infectious agents and infection-control procedures/protocols appropriate for and specific to their assigned duties (IB, IC).
2. Provide educational information appropriate in content and vocabulary to the educational level, literacy, and language of dental health-care personnel (IB, IC).

C. Immunization Programs

1. Develop a written comprehensive policy regarding immunizing dental health-care personnel, including a list of all required and recommended immunizations (IB).

2. Refer dental health-care personnel to a prearranged qualified health-care professional or to their own health-care professional to receive all appropriate immunizations based on the latest recommendations as well as their medical history and risk for occupational exposure (IB).

D. Exposure Prevention and Postexposure Management

1. Develop a comprehensive postexposure management and medical follow-up program (IB, IC).
   a. Include policies and procedures for prompt reporting, evaluation, counseling, treatment, and medical follow-up of occupational exposures.
   b. Establish mechanisms for referral to a qualified health-care professional for medical evaluation and follow-up.
   c. Conduct a baseline TST, preferably by using a two-step test, for all dental health-care personnel who might have contact with persons with suspected or confirmed infectious TB, regardless of the risk classification of the setting (IB).

E. Medical Conditions, Work-Related Illness, and Work Restrictions

1. Develop and have readily available to all dental health-care personnel comprehensive written policies regarding work restriction and exclusion that include a statement of authority defining who can implement such policies (IB).
2. Develop policies for work restriction and exclusion that encourage dental health-care personnel to seek appropriate preventive and curative care and report their illnesses, medical conditions, or treatments that can render them more susceptible to opportunistic infection or exposures; do not penalize dental health-care personnel with loss of wages, benefits, or job status (IB).

3. Develop policies and procedures for evaluation, diagnosis, and management of dental health-care personnel with suspected or known occupational contact dermatitis (IB).
4. Seek definitive diagnosis by a qualified health-care professional for any dental health-care personnel with suspected latex allergy to carefully determine its specific etiology and appropriate treatment as well as work restrictions and accommodations (IB).

F. Records Maintenance, Data Management, and Confidentiality

1. Establish and maintain confidential medical records (e.g., immunization records and documentation of tests received as a result of occupational exposure) for all dental health-care personnel (IB, IC).
2. Ensure that the practice complies with all applicable federal, state, and local laws regarding medical recordkeeping and confidentiality (IC).

II. Preventing Transmission of Bloodborne Pathogens

A. HBV Vaccination

1. Offer the HBV vaccination series to all dental health-care personnel with potential occupational exposure to blood or other potentially infectious material (IA, IC).
2. Always follow U.S. Public Health Service/CDC recommendations for hepatitis B vaccination, serologic testing, follow-up, and booster dosing (IA, IC).
3. Test dental health-care personnel for anti-HBs 1-2 months after completion of the 3-dose vaccination series (IA, IC).
4. Dental health-care personnel should complete a second 3-dose vaccine series or be evaluated to determine if they are HBsAg-positive if no antibody response occurs to the primary vaccine series (IA, IC).
5. Retest for anti-HBs at the completion of the second vaccine series. If no response to the second 3-dose series occurs, nonresponders should be tested for HBsAg (IC).
6. Counsel nonresponders to vaccination who are HBsAg-negative regarding their susceptibility to HBV infection and precautions to take (IA, IC).
7. Provide employees appropriate education regarding the risks of HBV transmission and the availability of the vaccine. Employees who decline the vaccination should sign a declination form to be kept on file with the employer (IC).

B. Preventing Exposures to Blood and Other Potentially Infectious Materials

1. General recommendations
   a. Use standard precautions (OSHA's [Occupational Safety and Health Administration's] bloodborne pathogen standard retains the term universal precautions) for all patient encounters (IA, IC).
   b. Consider sharp items (e.g., needles, scalers, burs, lab knives, and wires) that are contaminated with patient blood and saliva as potentially infective and establish engineering controls and work practices to prevent injuries (IB, IC).
   c. Implement a written, comprehensive program designed to minimize and manage dental health-care personnel exposures to blood and body fluids (IB, IC).
2. Engineering and work-practice controls
   a. Identify, evaluate, and select devices with engineered safety features at least annually and as they become available on the market (e.g., safer anesthetic syringes, blunt suture needle, retractable scalpel, or needleless IV systems) (IC).

   b. Place used disposable syringes and needles, scalpel blades, and other sharp items in appropriate puncture-resistant containers located as close as feasible to the area in which the items are used (IA, IC).
   c. Do not recap used needles by using both hands or any other technique that involves directing the point of a needle toward any part of the body. Do not bend, break, or remove needles before disposal (IA, IC).
   d. Use either a one-handed scoop technique or a mechanical device designed for holding the needle cap when recapping needles (e.g., between multiple injections and before removing from a nondisposable aspirating syringe) (IA, IC).
3. Postexposure management and prophylaxis
   a. Follow CDC recommendations after percutaneous, mucous membrane, or nonintact skin exposure to blood or other potentially infectious material (IA, IC).

III. Hand Hygiene

A. General Considerations

1. Perform hand hygiene with either a nonantimicrobial or antimicrobial soap and water when hands are visibly dirty or contaminated with blood or other potentially infectious material. If hands are not visibly soiled, an alcohol-based hand rub can also be used. Follow the manufacturer's instructions (IA).
2. Indications for hand hygiene include
   a. when hands are visibly soiled (IA, IC);
   b. after barehanded touching of inanimate objects likely to be contaminated by blood, saliva, or respiratory secretions (IA, IC);
   c. before and after treating each patient (IB);
   d. before donning gloves (IB); and
   e. immediately after removing gloves (IB, IC).
3. For oral surgical procedures, perform surgical hand antisepsis before donning sterile surgeon's gloves. Follow the manufacturer's instructions by using either an antimicrobial soap and water, or soap and water followed by drying hands and application of an alcohol-based surgical hand-scrub product with persistent activity (IB).
4. Store liquid hand-care products in either disposable closed containers or closed containers that can be washed and dried before refilling. Do not add soap or lotion to (i.e., top off) a partially empty dispenser (IA).

B. Special Considerations for Hand Hygiene and Glove Use

1. Use hand lotions to prevent skin dryness associated with handwashing (IA).
2. Consider the compatibility of lotion and antiseptic products and the effect of petroleum or other oil emollients on the integrity of gloves during product selection and glove use (IB).
3. Keep fingernails short with smooth, filed edges to allow thorough cleaning and prevent glove tears (II).
4. Do not wear artificial fingernails or extenders when having direct contact with patients at high risk (e.g., those in intensive care units or operating rooms) (IA).
5. Use of artificial fingernails is usually not recommended (II).
6. Do not wear hand or nail jewelry if it makes donning gloves more difficult or compromises the fit and integrity of the glove (II).

IV. PPE [Personal Protective Equipment]

A. Masks, Protective Eyewear, and Face Shields

1. Wear a surgical mask and eye protection with solid side

shields or a face shield to protect mucous membranes of the eyes, nose, and mouth during procedures likely to generate splashing or spattering of blood or other body fluids (IB, IC).

2. Change masks between patients or during patient treatment if the mask becomes wet (IB).

3. Clean with soap and water, or if visibly soiled, clean and disinfect reusable facial protective equipment (e.g., clinician and patient protective eyewear or face shields) between patients (II).

B. Protective Clothing

1. Wear protective clothing (e.g., reusable or disposable gown, laboratory coat, or uniform) that covers personal clothing and skin (e.g., forearms) likely to be soiled with blood, saliva, or other potentially infectious materials (IB, IC).

2. Change protective clothing if visibly soiled; change immediately or as soon as feasible if penetrated by blood or other potentially infectious fluids (IB, IC).

3. Remove barrier protection, including gloves, mask, eyewear, and gown before departing work area (e.g., dental patient care, instrument processing, or laboratory areas) (IC).

C. Gloves

1. Wear medical gloves when a potential exists for contacting blood, saliva, other potentially infectious materials (OPIM), or mucous membranes (IB, IC).

2. Wear a new pair of medical gloves for each patient, remove them promptly after use, and wash hands immediately to avoid transfer of microorganisms to other patients or environments (IB).

3. Remove gloves that are torn, cut, or punctured as soon as feasible and wash hands before regloving (IB, IC).

4. Do not wash surgeon's or patient examination gloves before use or wash, disinfect, or sterilize gloves for reuse (IB, IC).

5. Ensure that appropriate gloves in the correct size are readily accessible (IC).

6. Use appropriate gloves (e.g., puncture- and chemical-resistant utility gloves) when cleaning instruments and performing housekeeping tasks involving contact with blood or other potentially infectious materials (IB, IC).

7. Consult with glove manufacturers regarding the chemical compatibility of glove material and dental materials used (II).

D. Sterile Surgeon's Gloves and Double Gloving During Oral Surgical Procedures

1. Wear sterile surgeon's gloves when performing oral surgical procedures (IB).

2. No recommendation is offered regarding the effectiveness of wearing two pairs of gloves to prevent disease transmission during oral surgical procedures. The majority of studies among health-care personnel and dental health-care personnel have demonstrated a lower frequency of inner glove perforation and visible blood on the surgeon's hands when double gloves are worn; however, the effectiveness of wearing two pairs of gloves in preventing disease transmission has not been demonstrated (Unresolved issue).

V. Contact Dermatitis and Latex Hypersensitivity

A. General Recommendations

1. Educate dental health-care personnel regarding the signs, symptoms, and diagnoses of skin reactions associated with frequent hand hygiene and glove use (IB).

2. Screen all patients for latex allergy (e.g., take health history and refer for medical consultation when latex allergy is suspected) (IB).

3. Ensure a latex-safe environment for patients and dental health-care personnel with latex allergy (IB).

4. Have emergency treatment kits with latex-free products available at all times (II).

VI. Sterilization and Disinfection of Patient-Care Items

A. General Recommendations

1. Use only Food and Drug Administration-cleared medical devices for sterilization and follow the manufacturer's instructions for correct use (IB).

2. Clean and heat-sterilize critical dental instruments before each use (IA).

3. Clean and heat-sterilize semicritical items before each use (IB).

4. Allow packages to dry in the sterilizer before they are handled to avoid contamination (IB).

5. Use of heat-stable semicritical alternatives is encouraged (IB).

6. Reprocess heat-sensitive critical and semi-critical instruments by using FDA-cleared sterilant/high-level disinfectants or an FDA-cleared low-temperature sterilization method (e.g., ethylene oxide). Follow manufacturer's instructions for use of chemical sterilants/high-level disinfectants (IB).

7. Single-use disposable instruments are acceptable alternatives if they are used only once and disposed of correctly (IB, IC).

8. Do not use liquid chemical sterilants/high-level disinfectants for environmental surface disinfection or as holding solutions (IB, IC).

9. Ensure that noncritical patient-care items are barrier-protected or cleaned, or if visibly soiled, cleaned and disinfected after each use with an Environmental Protection Agency-registered hospital disinfectant. If visibly contaminated with blood, use an EPA-registered hospital disinfectant with a tuberculocidal claim (i.e., intermediate level) (IB).

10. Inform dental health-care personnel of all OSHA guidelines for exposure to chemical agents used for disinfection and sterilization. Using this report, identify areas and tasks that have potential for exposure (IC).

B. Instrument Processing Area

1. Designate a central processing area. Divide the instrument processing area, physically or, at a minimum, spatially, into distinct areas for 1) receiving, cleaning, and decontamination; 2) preparation and packaging; 3) sterilization; and 4) storage. Do not store instruments in an area where contaminated instruments are held or cleaned (II).

2. Train dental health-care personnel to employ work practices that prevent contamination of clean areas (II).

C. Receiving, Cleaning, and Decontamination Work Area

1. Minimize handling of loose contaminated instruments during transport to the instrument processing area. Use work-practice controls (e.g., carry instruments in a covered container) to minimize exposure potential (II). Clean all visible blood and other contamination from dental instruments and devices before sterilization or disinfection procedures (IA).

2. Use automated cleaning equipment (e.g., ultrasonic cleaner or washer-disinfector) to remove debris to improve cleaning effectiveness and decrease worker exposure to blood (IB).

3. Use work-practice controls that minimize contact with sharp instruments if manual cleaning is necessary (e.g., long-handled brush) (IC).

4. Wear puncture- and chemical-resistant/heavy-duty utility gloves for instrument cleaning and decontamination procedures (IB).

5. Wear appropriate PPE (e.g., mask, protective eyewear, and gown) when splashing or spraying is anticipated during cleaning (IC).

D. Preparation and Packaging

1. Use an internal chemical indicator in each package. If the internal indicator cannot be seen from outside the package, also use an external indicator (II).

2. Use a container system or wrapping compatible with the type of sterilization process used and that has received FDA clearance (IB).

3. Before sterilization of critical and semicritical instruments, inspect instruments for cleanliness, then wrap or place them in containers designed to maintain sterility during storage (e.g., cassettes and organizing trays) (IA).

E. Sterilization of Unwrapped Instruments

1. Clean and dry instruments before the unwrapped sterilization cycle (IB).

2. Use mechanical and chemical indicators for each unwrapped sterilization cycle (i.e., place an internal chemical indicator among the instruments or items to be sterilized) (IB).

3. Allow unwrapped instruments to dry and cool in the sterilizer before they are handled to avoid contamination and thermal injury (II).

4. Semicritical instruments that will be used immediately or within a short time can be sterilized unwrapped on a tray or in a container system, provided that the instruments are handled aseptically during removal from the sterilizer and transport to the point of use (II).

5. Critical instruments intended for immediate reuse can be sterilized unwrapped if the instruments are maintained sterile during removal from the sterilizer and transport to the point of use (e.g., transported in a sterile covered container) (IB).

6. Do not sterilize implantable devices unwrapped (IB).

7. Do not store critical instruments unwrapped (IB).

F. Sterilization Monitoring

1. Use mechanical, chemical, and biological monitors according to the manufacturer's instructions to ensure the effectiveness of the sterilization process (IB).

2. Monitor each load with mechanical (e.g., time, temperature, and pressure) and chemical indicators (II).

3. Place a chemical indicator on the inside of each package. If the internal indicator is not visible from the outside, also place an exterior chemical indicator on the package (II).

4. Place items/packages correctly and loosely into the sterilizer so as not to impede penetration of the sterilant (IB).

5. Do not use instrument packs if mechanical or chemical indicators indicate inadequate processing (IB).

6. Monitor sterilizers at least weekly by using a biological indicator with a matching control (i.e., biological indicator and control from same lot number) (IB).

7. Use a biological indicator for every sterilizer load that contains an implantable device. Verify results before using the implantable device, whenever possible (IB).

8. The following are recommended in the case of a positive spore test:
   a. Remove the sterilizer from service and review sterilization procedures (e.g., work practices and use of mechanical and chemical indicators) to determine whether operator error could be responsible (II).
   b. Retest the sterilizer by using biological, mechanical, and chemical indicators after correcting any identified procedural problems (II).
   c. If the repeat spore test is negative, and mechanical and chemical indicators are within normal limits, put the sterilizer back in service (II).

9. The following are recommended if the repeat spore test is positive:
   a. Do not use the sterilizer until it has been inspected or repaired or the exact reason for the positive test has been determined (II).
   b. Recall, to the extent possible, and reprocess all items processed since the last negative spore test (II).
   c. Before placing the sterilizer back in service, rechallenge the sterilizer with biological indicator tests in three consecutive empty chamber sterilization cycles after the cause of the sterilizer failure has been determined and corrected (II).

10. Maintain sterilization records (i.e., mechanical, chemical, and biological) in compliance with state and local regulations (IB).

G. Storage Area for Sterilized Items and Clean Dental Supplies

1. Implement practices on the basis of date- or event-related shelf-life for storage of wrapped, sterilized instruments and devices (IB).

2. Even for event-related packaging, at a minimum, place the date of sterilization, and if multiple sterilizers are used in the facility, the sterilizer used, on the outside of the packaging material to facilitate the retrieval of processed items in the event of a sterilization failure (IB).

3. Examine wrapped packages of sterilized instruments before opening them to ensure the barrier wrap has not been compromised during storage (II).

4. Reclean, repack, and resterilize any instrument package that has been compromised (II).

5. Store sterile items and dental supplies in covered or closed cabinets, if possible (II).

VII. Environmental Infection Control

A. General Recommendations

1. Follow the manufacturers' instructions for correct use of cleaning and EPA-registered hospital disinfecting products (IB, IC).

2. Do not use liquid chemical sterilants/high-level disinfectants for disinfection of environmental surfaces (clinical contact or housekeeping) (IB, IC).

3. Use PPE, as appropriate, when cleaning and disinfecting

environmental surfaces. Such equipment might include gloves (e.g., puncture- and chemical-resistant utility), protective clothing (e.g., gown, jacket, or lab coat), and protective eyewear/face shield, and mask (IC).

B. Clinical Contact Surfaces

1. Use surface barriers to protect clinical contact surfaces, particularly those that are difficult to clean (e.g., switches on dental chairs) and change surface barriers between patients (II).

2. Clean and disinfect clinical contact surfaces that are not barrier-protected, by using an EPA-registered hospital disinfectant with a low- (i.e., HIV and HBV label claims) to intermediate-level (i.e., tuberculocidal claim) activity after each patient. Use an intermediate-level disinfectant if visibly contaminated with blood (IB).

C. Housekeeping Surfaces

1. Clean housekeeping surfaces (e.g., floors, walls, and sinks) with a detergent and water or an EPA-registered hospital disinfectant/detergent on a routine basis, depending on the nature of the surface and type and degree of contamination, and as appropriate, based on the location in the facility, and when visibly soiled (IB).

2. Clean mops and cloths after use and allow to dry before reuse; or use single-use, disposable mop heads or cloths (II).

3. Prepare fresh cleaning or EPA-registered disinfecting solutions daily and as instructed by the manufacturer. (II).

4. Clean walls, blinds, and window curtains in patient-care areas when they are visibly dusty or soiled (II).

D. Spills of Blood and Body Substances

1. Clean spills of blood or other potentially infectious materials and decontaminate surface with an EPA-registered hospital disinfectant with low- (i.e., HBV and HIV label claims) to intermediate-level (i.e., tuberculocidal claim) activity, depending on size of spill and surface porosity (IB, IC).

E. Carpet and Cloth Furnishings

1. Avoid using carpeting and cloth-upholstered furnishings in dental operatories, laboratories, and instrument processing areas (II).

F. Regulated Medical Waste

1. General Recommendations

a. Develop a medical waste management program. Disposal of regulated medical waste must follow federal, state, and local regulations (IC).

b. Ensure that dental health-care personnel who handle and dispose of regulated medical waste are trained in appropriate handling and disposal methods and informed of the possible health and safety hazards (IC).

2. Management of Regulated Medical Waste in Dental Health-Care Facilities

a. Use a color-coded or labeled container that prevents leakage (e.g., biohazard bag) to contain nonsharp regulated medical waste (IC).

b. Place sharp items (e.g., needles, scalpel blades, orthodontic bands, broken metal instruments, and burs) in an appropriate sharps container (e.g., puncture resistant, color-coded, and leakproof). Close container immediately before removal or replacement to prevent spillage or protrusion of contents during handling, storage, transport, or shipping (IC).

c. Pour blood, suctioned fluids or other liquid waste carefully into a drain connected to a sanitary sewer system, if local sewage discharge requirements are met and the state has declared this an acceptable method of disposal. Wear appropriate PPE while performing this task (IC).

VIII. Dental Unit Waterlines, Biofilm, and Water Quality

A. General Recommendations

1. Use water that meets EPA regulatory standards for drinking water (i.e., <500 CFU/mL of heterotrophic water bacteria) for routine dental treatment output water (IB, IC).

2. Consult with the dental unit manufacturer for appropriate methods and equipment to maintain the recommended quality of dental water (II).

3. Follow recommendations for monitoring water quality provided by the manufacturer of the unit or waterline treatment product (II).

4. Discharge water and air for a minimum of 20-30 seconds after each patient, from any device connected to the dental water system that enters the patient's mouth (e.g., handpieces, ultrasonic scalers, and air/water syringes) (II).

5. Consult with the dental unit manufacturer on the need for periodic maintenance of antiretraction mechanisms (IB).

B. Boil-Water Advisories

1. The following apply while a boil-water advisory is in effect:

a. Do not deliver water from the public water system to the patient through the dental operative unit, ultrasonic scaler, or other dental equipment that uses the public water system (IB, IC).

b. Do not use water from the public water system for dental treatment, patient rinsing, or handwashing (IB, IC).

c. For handwashing, use antimicrobial-containing products that do not require water for use (e.g., alcohol-based hand rubs). If hands are visibly contaminated, use bottled water, if available, and soap for handwashing or an antiseptic towelette (IB, IC).

2. The following apply when the boil-water advisory is cancelled:

a. Follow guidance given by the local water utility regarding adequate flushing of waterlines. If no guidance is provided, flush dental waterlines and faucets for 1-5 minutes before using for patient care (IC).

b. Disinfect dental waterlines as recommended by the dental unit manufacturer (II).

IX. Special Considerations

A. Dental Handpieces and Other Devices Attached to Air and Waterlines

1. Clean and heat-sterilize handpieces and other intraoral instruments that can be removed from the air and waterlines of dental units between patients (IB, IC).

2. Follow the manufacturer's instructions for cleaning, lubrication, and sterilization of handpieces and other intraoral instruments that can be removed from the air and waterlines of dental units (IB).

3. Do not surface-disinfect, use liquid chemical sterilants, or ethylene oxide on handpieces and other intraoral instruments that can be removed from the air and waterlines of dental units (IC).

4. Do not advise patients to close their lips tightly around the tip of the saliva ejector to evacuate oral fluids (II).

B. Dental Radiology

1. Wear gloves when exposing radiographs and handling contaminated film packets. Use other PPE (e.g., protective eyewear, mask, and gown) as appropriate if spattering of blood or other body fluids is likely (IA, IC).

2. Use heat-tolerant or disposable intraoral devices whenever possible (e.g., film-holding and positioning devices). Clean and heat-sterilize heat-tolerant devices between patients. At a minimum, high-level disinfect semicritical heat-sensitive devices, according to manufacturer's instructions (IB).

3. Transport and handle exposed radiographs in an aseptic manner to prevent contamination of developing equipment (II).

4. The following apply for digital radiography sensors:
   a. Use FDA-cleared barriers (IB).
   b. Clean and heat-sterilize, or high-level disinfect, between patients, barrier-protected semicritical items. If the item cannot tolerate these procedures then, at a minimum, protect with an FDA-cleared barrier and clean and disinfect with an EPA-registered hospital disinfectant with intermediate-level (i.e., tuberculocidal claim) activity, between patients. Consult with the manufacturer for methods of disinfection and sterilization of digital radiology sensors and for protection of associated computer hardware (IB).

C. Aseptic Technique for Parenteral Medications

1. Do not administer medication from a syringe to multiple patients, even if the needle on the syringe is changed (IA).

2. Use single-dose vials for parenteral medications when possible (II).

3. Do not combine the leftover contents of single-use vials for later use (IA).

4. The following apply if multidose vials are used:
   a. Cleanse the access diaphragm with 70% alcohol before inserting a device into the vial (IA).
   b. Use a sterile device to access a multiple-dose vial and avoid touching the access diaphragm. Both the needle and syringe used to access the multidose vial should be sterile. Do not reuse a syringe even if the needle is changed (IA).
   c. Keep multidose vials away from the immediate patient treatment area to prevent inadvertent contamination by spray or spatter (II).
   d. Discard the multidose vial if sterility is compromised (IA).

5. Use fluid infusion and administration sets (i.e., IV bags, tubings and connections) for one patient only and dispose of appropriately (IB).

D. Single-Use (Disposable) Devices

1. Use single-use devices for one patient only and dispose of them appropriately (IC).

E. Preprocedural Mouth Rinses

1. No recommendation is offered regarding use of preprocedural antimicrobial mouth rinses to prevent clinical infections among dental health-care personnel or patients. Although studies have demonstrated that a preprocedural antimicrobial rinse (e.g., chlorhexidine gluconate, essential oils, or povidone-iodine) can reduce the level of oral microorganisms in aerosols and spatter generated during routine dental procedures and can decrease the number of microorganisms introduced in the patient's bloodstream during invasive dental procedures, the scientific evidence is inconclusive that using these rinses prevents clinical infections among dental health-care personnel or patients (see discussion, Preprocedural Mouth Rinses) (Unresolved issue).

F. Oral Surgical Procedures

1. The following apply when performing oral surgical procedures:
   a. Perform surgical hand antisepsis by using an antimicrobial product (e.g., antimicrobial soap and water, or soap and water followed by alcohol-based hand scrub with persistent activity) before donning sterile surgeon's gloves (IB).
   b. Use sterile surgeon's gloves (IB).
   c. Use sterile saline or sterile water as a coolant/irrigant when performing oral surgical procedures. Use devices specifically designed for delivering sterile irrigating fluids (e.g., bulb syringe, single-use disposable products, and sterilizable tubing).

G. Handling of Biopsy Specimens

1. During transport, place biopsy specimens in a sturdy, leakproof container labeled with the biohazard symbol (IC).

2. If a biopsy specimen container is visibly contaminated, clean and disinfect the outside of a container or place it in an impervious bag labeled with the biohazard symbol (IC).

H. Handling of Extracted Teeth

1. Dispose of extracted teeth as regulated medical waste unless returned to the patient (IC).

2. Do not dispose of extracted teeth containing amalgam in regulated medical waste intended for incineration (II).

3. Clean and place extracted teeth in a leakproof container, labeled with a biohazard symbol, and maintain hydration for transport to educational institutions or a dental laboratory (IC).

4. Heat-sterilize teeth that do not contain amalgam before they are used for educational purposes (IB).

I. Dental Laboratory

1. Use PPE when handling items received in the laboratory until they have been decontaminated (IA, IC).

2. Before they are handled in the laboratory, clean, disinfect, and rinse all dental prostheses and prosthodontic materials (e.g., impressions, bite registrations, occlusal rims, and extracted teeth) by using an EPA-registered hospital disinfectant having at least an intermediate-level (i.e., tuberculocidal claim) activity (IB).

3. Consult with manufacturers regarding the stability of specific materials (e.g., impression materials) relative to disinfection procedures (II).

4. Include specific information regarding disinfection techniques used (e.g., solution used and duration), when laboratory cases are sent off-site and on their return (II).

5. Clean and heat-sterilize heat-tolerant items used in the mouth (e.g., metal impression trays and face-bow forks) (IB).

6. Follow manufacturers' instructions for cleaning and sterilizing or disinfecting items that become contaminated but do not normally contact the patient (e.g., burs, polishing points, rag wheels, articulators, case pans, and lathes). If manufacturer instructions are unavailable, clean and heat-sterilize heat-tolerant items or clean and disinfect with an EPA-registered hospital disinfectant with low- (HIV, HBV effectiveness claim) to intermediate-level (tuberculocidal

claim) activity, depending on the degree of contamination (II).

J. Laser/Electrosurgery Plumes/Surgical Smoke

1. No recommendation is offered regarding practices to reduce dental health-care personnel exposure to laser plumes/surgical smoke when using lasers in dental practice. Practices to reduce health-care personnel exposure to laser plumes/surgical smoke have been suggested, including use of a) standard precautions (e.g., high-filtration surgical masks and possibly full face shields); b) central room suction units with in-line filters to collect particulate matter from minimal plumes; and c) dedicated mechanical smoke exhaust systems with a high-efficiency filter to remove substantial amounts of laser-plume particles. The effect of the exposure (e.g., disease transmission or adverse respiratory effects) on dental health-care personnel from dental applications of lasers has not been adequately evaluated (see previous discussion, Laser/Electrosurgery Plumes or Surgical Smoke [in the complete CDC document]) (Unresolved issue).

K. *Mycobacterium tuberculosis*

1. General Recommendations
   a. Educate all dental health-care personnel regarding the recognition of signs, symptoms, and transmission of TB [tuberculosis] (IB).
   b. Conduct a baseline TST [tuberculin skin test], preferably by using a two-step test, for all dental health-care personnel who might have contact with persons with suspected or confirmed active TB, regardless of the risk classification of the setting (IB).
   c. Assess each patient for a history of TB as well as symptoms indicative of TB and document on the medical history form (IB).
   d. Follow CDC recommendations for 1) developing, maintaining, and implementing a written TB infection-control plan; 2) managing a patient with suspected or active TB; 3) completing a community risk-assessment to guide employee TSTs and follow-up; and 4) managing dental health-care personnel with TB disease (IB).
2. The following apply for patients known or suspected to have active TB:
   a. Evaluate the patient away from other patients and dental health-care personnel. When not being evaluated, the patient should wear a surgical mask or be instructed to cover mouth and nose when coughing or sneezing (IB).
   b. Defer elective dental treatment until the patient is non-infectious (IB).
   c. Refer patients requiring urgent dental treatment to a previously identified facility with TB engineering controls and a respiratory protection program (IB).

L. Creutzfeldt-Jakob Disease (CJD) and Other Prion Diseases

1. No recommendation is offered regarding use of special precautions in addition to standard precautions when treating known CJD or vCJD patients. Potential infectivity of oral tissues in CJD or vCJD patients is an unresolved issue. Scientific data indicate the risk, if any, of sporadic CJD transmission during dental and oral surgical procedures is low to nil. Until additional information exists regarding the transmissibility of CJD or vCJD during dental procedures, special precautions in addition to standard precautions might be indicated when treating known CJD or vCJD patients; a list of such precautions is provided for consideration without recommendation (see Creutzfeldt-Jakob Disease and Other Prion Diseases [in the complete CDC document]) (Unresolved issue).

M. PROGRAM EVALUATION

1. Establish routine evaluation of the infection-control program, including evaluation of performance indicators, at an established frequency (II).

Infection Prevention Checklist for Dental Settings:
Basic Expectations for Safe Care

The following is a companion to the *Summary of Infection Prevention in Dental Settings: Basic Expectations for Safe Care.* The checklist should be used –

1. To ensure the dental health care setting has appropriate infection prevention policies and practices in place, including appropriate training and education of dental health care personnel (DHCP) on infection prevention practices, and adequate supplies to allow DHCP to provide safe care and a safe working environment.

2. To systematically assess personnel compliance with the expected infection prevention practices and to provide feedback to DHCP regarding performance. Assessment of compliance should be conducted by direct observation of DHCP during the performance of their duties.

DHCP using this checklist should identify all procedures performed in their setting and refer to appropriate sections of this checklist to conduct their evaluation. Certain sections may not apply (e.g., some settings may not perform surgical procedures or use medications in vials, such as for conscious sedation). If the answer to any of the applicable listed questions is no, efforts should be made to determine why the correct practice was not being performed, correct the practice, educate DHCP (if applicable), and reassess the practice to ensure compliance. Consideration should also be made to determine the risk posed to patients by the deficient practice. Certain infection prevention and control lapses (e.g., re-use of syringes on more than one patient, sterilization failures) can result in bloodborne pathogen transmission and measures to address the lapses should be taken immediately. Identification of such lapses may warrant immediate consultation with the state or local health department and appropriate notification and testing of potentially affected patients.

Section I lists administrative policies and dental setting practices that should be included in the site-specific written infection prevention and control program with supportive documentation. Section II describes personnel compliance with infection prevention and control practices that fulfill the expectations for dental health care settings. This checklist can serve as an evaluation tool to monitor DHCP compliance with the CDC's recommendations and provide an assurance of quality control.

Infection Prevention Checklist
Section I. Policies and Practices

Facility Name: _____

Completed by: _____

Date: _____

I.1 Administrative Measures

Elements To Be Assessed	Assessment	Notes/Areas For Improvement
A. Written infection prevention policies and procedures specific for the dental setting are available, current, and based on evidence-based guidelines (e.g., CDC / Healthcare Infection Control Practices Advisory Committee [HICPAC]), regulations, or standards **Note:** *Policies and procedures should be appropriate for the services provided by the dental setting and should extend beyond the Occupational Safety and Health Administration (OSHA) bloodborne pathogens training.*	☐ Yes ☐ No	
B. Infection prevention policies and procedures are reassessed at least annually or according to state or federal requirements, and updated if appropriate **Note:** *This may be performed during the required annual review of the dental setting's OSHA Exposure Control Plan.*	☐ Yes ☐ No	
C. At least one individual trained in infection prevention is assigned responsibility for coordinating the program	☐ Yes ☐ No	
D. Supplies necessary for adherence to Standard Precautions are readily available **Note:** *This includes, but is not limited to hand hygiene products, safer devices to reduce percutaneous injuries, and personal protective equipment (PPE).*	☐ Yes ☐ No	
E. Facility has system for early detection and management of potentially infectious persons at initial points of patient encounter **Note:** *System may include taking a travel and occupational history, as appropriate, and elements described under respiratory hygiene / cough etiquette.*	☐ Yes ☐ No	

continued on next page

I.2 Infection Prevention Education and Training

Elements To Be Assessed	Assessment	Notes/Areas For Improvement

A. DHCP receive job or task-specific training on infection prevention policies and procedures and the OSHA bloodborne pathogens standard —
     a. upon hire
     b. annually
     c. when new tasks or procedures affect the
        employee's occupational exposure
     d. according to state or federal requirements
 	
 Note: *This includes those employed by outside agencies and available by contract or on a volunteer basis to the dental setting.*
	☐ Yes ☐ No
	 ☐ Yes ☐ No
	 ☐ Yes ☐ No
	
	 ☐ Yes ☐ No	

B. Training records are maintained in accordance with state and federal requirements	☐ Yes ☐ No	

I.3 Dental Healthcare Personnel Safety

Elements To Be Assessed	Assessment	Notes/Areas For Improvement
A. Facility has an exposure control plan that is tailored to the specific requirements of the facility (e.g., addresses potential hazards posed by specific services provided by the facility) *Note:* *A model template that includes a guide for creating an exposure control plan that meets the requirements of the OSHA Bloodborne Pathogens Standard is available at: www.osha.gov/Publications/osha3186.pdf.*	☐ Yes ☐ No	

B. DHCP for whom contact with blood or OPIM is anticipated are trained on the OSHA Bloodborne Pathogens Standard:
     a. upon hire
     b. at least annually
	☐ Yes ☐ No
	 ☐ Yes ☐ No	

C. Current CDC recommendations for immunizations, evaluation, and follow-up are available. There is a written policy regarding immunizing DHCP, including a list of all required and recommended immunizations for DHCP (e.g., hepatitis B, MMR (measles , mumps, rubella), varicella (chickenpox), Tdap (tetanus, diphtheria, pertussis)	☐ Yes ☐ No	
D Hepatitis B vaccination is available at no cost to all employees who are at risk of occupational exposure to blood or other potentially infectious material (OPIM)	☐ Yes ☐ No	
E. Post-vaccination screening for protective levels of hepatitis B surface antibody is conducted 1-2 months after completion of the 3-dose vaccination series	☐ Yes ☐ No	
F. All DHCP are offered annual influenza vaccination *Note:* *Providing the vaccination at no cost is a strategy that may increase use of this preventive service.*	☐ Yes ☐ No	

continued on next page

I.3 Dental Health Care Personnel Safety

Elements To Be Assessed	Assessment	Notes/Areas For Improvement
G. All DHCP receive baseline tuberculosis (TB) screening upon hire regardless of the risk classification of the setting	☐ Yes ☐ No	
H. A log of needlesticks, sharps injuries, and other employee exposure events is maintained according to state or federal requirements	☐ Yes ☐ No	
I. Referral arrangements are in place to qualified health care professionals (e.g., occupational health program of a hospital, educational institutions, health care facilities that offer personnel health services) to ensure prompt and appropriate provision of preventive services, occupationally-related medical services, and postexposure management with medical follow-up	☐ Yes ☐ No	
J. Following an occupational exposure event, postexposure evaluation and follow-up, including prophylaxis as appropriate, are available at no cost to employee and are supervised by a qualified health care professional	☐ Yes ☐ No	
K. Facility has well-defined policies concerning contact of personnel with patients when personnel have potentially transmissible conditions. These policies include —		
a. work-exclusion policies that encourage reporting of illnesses and do not penalize staff with loss of wages, benefits, or job status	☐ Yes ☐ No	
b. education of personnel on the importance of prompt reporting of illness to supervisor	☐ Yes ☐ No	

I.4 Program Evaluation

Elements To Be Assessed	Assessment	Notes/Areas For Improvement
A. Written policies and procedures for routine monitoring and evaluation of the infection prevention and control program are available	☐ Yes ☐ No	
B. Adherence with certain practices such as immunizations, hand hygiene, sterilization monitoring, and proper use of PPE is monitored and feedback is provided to DHCP	☐ Yes ☐ No	

I.5 Hand Hygiene

Elements To Be Assessed	Assessment	Notes/Areas For Improvement
A. Supplies necessary for adherence to hand hygiene for routine dental procedures (e.g., soap, water, paper towels, alcohol-based hand rub) are readily accessible to DHCP	☐ Yes ☐ No	
a. if surgical procedures are performed, appropriate supplies are available for surgical hand scrub technique (e.g., antimicrobial soap, alcohol based hand scrub with persistent activity)	☐ Yes ☐ No	

Note: *Examples of surgical procedures include biopsy, periodontal surgery, apical surgery, implant surgery, and surgical extractions of teeth.*

continued on next page

I.5 Hand Hygiene

Elements To Be Assessed	Assessment	Notes/Areas For Improvement
B. DHCP are trained regarding appropriate indications for hand hygiene including handwashing, hand anti-sepsis, and surgical hand antisepsis **Note:** *Use soap and water when hands are visibly soiled (e.g., blood, body fluids). Alcohol-based hand rub may be used in all other situations.*	☐ Yes ☐ No	

I.6 Personal Protective Equipment (PPE)

Elements To Be Assessed	Assessment	Notes/Areas For Improvement
A. Sufficient and appropriate PPE is available (e.g., examination gloves, surgical face masks, protective clothing, protective eyewear / face shields, utility gloves, sterile surgeon's gloves for surgical procedures) and readily accessible to DHCP	☐ Yes ☐ No	
B. DHCP receive training on proper selection and use of PPE	☐ Yes ☐ No	

I.7 Respiratory Hygiene / Cough Etiquette

Elements To Be Assessed	Assessment	Notes/Areas For Improvement
A. Policies and procedures to contain respiratory secretions in people who have signs and symptoms of a respiratory infection, beginning at point of entry to the dental setting have been implemented. Measures include —		
a. posting signs at entrances (with instructions to patients with symptoms of respiratory infection to cover their mouths / noses when coughing or sneezing, use and dispose of tissues, and perform hand hygiene after hands have been in contact with respiratory secretions)	☐ Yes ☐ No	
b. providing tissues and no-touch receptacles for disposal of tissues	☐ Yes ☐ No	
c. providing resources for patients to perform hand hygiene in or near waiting areas	☐ Yes ☐ No	
d. offering face masks to coughing patients and other symptomatic persons when they enter the setting	☐ Yes ☐ No	
e. providing space and encouraging persons with respiratory symptoms to sit as far away from others as possible — if possible, a separate waiting area is ideal	☐ Yes ☐ No	
B. DHCP receive training on the importance of containing respiratory secretions in people who have signs and symptoms of a respiratory infection	☐ Yes ☐ No	

I.8 Sharps Safety

Elements To Be Assessed	Assessment	Notes/Areas For Improvement
A. Written policies, procedures, and guidelines for exposure prevention and postexposure management are available	☐ Yes ☐ No	

continued on next page

I.8 Sharps Safety

Elements To Be Assessed	Assessment	Notes/Areas For Improvement
B. DHCP identify, evaluate, and select devices with engineered safety features (e.g., safer anesthetic syringes, blunt suture needle, safety scalpels, or needleless IV systems) — a. at least annually b. as they become available in the market **Note::** *If staff inquire about the availability of new safety devices or safer options and find none are available, DHCP can document these findings in their office exposure control plan.*	☐ Yes ☐ No ☐ Yes ☐ No	

I.9 Safe Injection Practices

Elements To Be Assessed	Assessment	Notes/Areas For Improvement
A. Written policies, procedures, and guidelines for safe injection practices (e.g., aseptic technique for parenteral medications) are available	☐ Yes ☐ No	
B. Injections are required to be prepared using aseptic technique in a clean area free from contamination or contact with blood, body fluids, or contaminated equipment	☐ Yes ☐ No	

I.10 Sterilization and Disinfection of Patient-Care Items and Devices

Elements To Be Assessed	Assessment	Notes/Areas For Improvement
A. Written policies and procedures are available to ensure reusable patient care instruments and devices are cleaned and reprocessed appropriately before use on another patient	☐ Yes ☐ No	
B. Policies, procedures, and manufacturer reprocessing instructions for reusable instruments and dental devices are available, ideally in or near the reprocessing areas	☐ Yes ☐ No	
C. DHCP responsible for reprocessing reusable dental instruments and devices are appropriately trained — a. upon hire b. at least annually c. whenever new equipment or processes are introduced	☐ Yes ☐ No ☐ Yes ☐ No ☐ Yes ☐ No	
D. Training and equipment are available to ensure that DHCP wear appropriate PPE (e.g., examination or heavy duty utility gloves, protective clothing, masks, eye protection) to prevent exposure to infectious agents or chemicals **Note:** *The exact type of PPE depends on infectious or chemical agent and anticipated type of exposure*	☐ Yes ☐ No	
E. Routine maintenance for sterilization equipment is: a. performed according to manufacturer instructions b. documented by written maintenance records	☐ Yes ☐ No ☐ Yes ☐ No	

continued on next page

I.10 Sterilization and Disinfection of Patient-Care Items and Devices

Elements To Be Assessed	Assessment	Notes/Areas For Improvement
F. Policies and procedures are in place outlining dental setting response (e.g., recall of device, risk assessment) in the event of a reprocessing error / failure	☐ Yes ☐ No	

I.11 Environmental Infection Prevention and Control

Elements To Be Assessed	Assessment	Notes/Areas For Improvement
A. Written policies and procedures are available for routine cleaning and disinfection of environmental surfaces (i.e., clinical contact and housekeeping)	☐ Yes ☐ No	
B. DHCP performing environmental infection prevention procedures receive job-specific training about infection prevention and control management of clinical contact and housekeeping surfaces — a. upon hire b. when procedures/policies change c. at least annually	☐ Yes ☐ No ☐ Yes ☐ No ☐ Yes ☐ No	
C. Training and equipment are available to ensure that DHCP wear appropriate PPE (e.g., examination or heavy duty utility gloves, protective clothing, masks, and eye protection) to prevent exposure to infectious agents or chemicals	☐ Yes ☐ No	
D. Cleaning, disinfection and use of surface barriers are periodically monitored and evaluated to ensure that they are consistently and correctly performed	☐ Yes ☐ No	
E. Procedures are in place for decontamination of spills of blood or other body fluids	☐ Yes ☐ No	

I.12 Dental Unit Water Quality

Elements To Be Assessed	Assessment	Notes/Areas For Improvement
A. Policies and procedures are in place for maintaining dental unit water quality that meets Environmental Protection Agency (EPA) regulatory standards for drinking water (i.e., ≤ 500 CFU / mL of heterotrophic water bacteria) for routine dental treatment output water	☐ Yes ☐ No	
B: Policies and procedures are in place for using sterile water as a coolant / irrigant when performing surgical procedures *Note: Examples of surgical procedures include biopsy, periodontal surgery, apical surgery, implant surgery, and surgical extractions of teeth.*	☐ Yes ☐ No	
C. Written policies and procedures are available outlining response to a community boil-water advisory	☐ Yes ☐ No	

Section II: Direct Observation of Personnel and Patient-Care Practices

Facility Name: _____

Completed by: _____

Date: _____

II.1 Hand Hygiene is Performed Correctly

Elements To Be Assessed	Assessment	Notes/Areas For Improvement
A. When hands are visibly soiled	☐ Yes ☐ No	
B. After barehanded touching of instruments, equipment, materials and other objects likely to be contaminated by blood, saliva, or respiratory secretions	☐ Yes ☐ No	
C. Before and after treating each patient	☐ Yes ☐ No	
D. Before putting on gloves	☐ Yes ☐ No	
E. Immediately after removing gloves	☐ Yes ☐ No	
F. Surgical hand scrub is performed before putting on sterile surgeon's gloves for all surgical procedures **Note:** *Examples of surgical procedures include biopsy, periodontal surgery, apical surgery, implant surgery, and surgical extractions of teeth.*	☐ Yes ☐ No	

II.2 Personal Protective Equipment (PPE) is Used Correctly

Elements To Be Assessed	Assessment	Notes/Areas For Improvement
A. PPE is removed before leaving the work area (e.g., dental patient care, instrument processing, or laboratory areas)	☐ Yes ☐ No	
B. Hand hygiene is performed immediately after removal of PPE	☐ Yes ☐ No	
C. Masks, Protective Eyewear, and Face Shields		
a. DHCP wear surgical masks during procedures that are likely to generate splashes or sprays of blood or other body fluids	☐ Yes ☐ No	
b. DHCP wear eye protection with solid side shields or a face shield during procedures that are likely to generate splashes or sprays of blood or other body fluids	☐ Yes ☐ No	
c. DHCP change masks between patients and during patient treatment if the mask becomes wet	☐ Yes ☐ No	

continued on next page

II.2 Personal Protective Equipment (PPE) is Used Correctly

Elements To Be Assessed	Assessment	Notes/Areas For Improvement
D. Gloves		
a. DHCP wear gloves for potential contact with blood, body fluids, mucous membranes, non-intact skin, or contaminated equipment	☐ Yes ☐ No	
b. DHCP change gloves between patients; do not wear the same pair of gloves for the care of more than one patient	☐ Yes ☐ No	
c. DHCP do not wash examination or sterile surgeon's gloves for the purpose of reuse	☐ Yes ☐ No	
d. DHCP wear puncture- and chemical-resistant utility gloves when cleaning instruments and performing housekeeping tasks involving contact with blood or OPIM	☐ Yes ☐ No	
e. DHCP wear sterile surgeon's gloves for all surgical procedures ***Note:*** *Examples of surgical procedures include biopsy, periodontal surgery, apical surgery, implant surgery, and surgical extractions of teeth.*	☐ Yes ☐ No	
f. DHCP remove gloves that are torn, cut, or punctured and perform hand hygiene before putting on new gloves	☐ Yes ☐ No	
E. Protective Clothing		
a. DHCP wear protective clothing (e.g., reusable or disposable gown, laboratory coat, or uniform) that covers personal clothing and skin (e.g., forearms) likely to be soiled with blood, saliva, or OPIM	☐ Yes ☐ No	
b. DHCP change protective clothing if visibly soiled and immediately or as soon as possible if penetrated by blood or other potentially infectious fluids	☐ Yes ☐ No	

II.3 Respiratory Hygiene/Cough Etiquette

Elements To Be Assessed	Assessment	Notes/Areas For Improvement
A. Signs are posted at entrances (with instructions to patients with symptoms of respiratory infection to cover their mouths / noses when coughing or sneezing, use and dispose of tissues, and perform hand hygiene after hands have been in contact with respiratory secretions)	☐ Yes ☐ No	
B. Tissues and no-touch receptacles for disposal of tissues are provided	☐ Yes ☐ No	
C. Resources are provided for patients to perform hand hygiene in or near waiting areas	☐ Yes ☐ No	
D. Face masks are offered to coughing patients and other symptomatic persons when they enter the setting	☐ Yes ☐ No	
E. Persons with respiratory symptoms are encouraged to sit as far away from others as possible. If possible, a separate waiting area is ideal	☐ Yes ☐ No	

continued on next page

Section II. Direct Observation of Personnel and Patient-care Practices

II.4 Sharps Safety

Elements To Be Assessed	Assessment	Notes/Areas For Improvement
A. Engineering controls (e.g., self-sheathing anesthetic needles, safety scalpels, needleless IV ports) are used to prevent injuries	☐ Yes ☐ No	
B. Work practice controls (e.g., one-handed scoop technique for recapping needles, removing burs before disconnecting handpieces) are used to prevent injuries	☐ Yes ☐ No	
C. DHCP do not recap used needles by using both hands or any other technique that involves directing the point of a needle toward any part of the body	☐ Yes ☐ No	
D. DHCP use either a one-handed scoop technique or a mechanical device designed for holding the needle cap when recapping needles (e.g., between multiple injections and before removing from a reusable aspirating syringe)	☐ Yes ☐ No	
E. All sharps are disposed of in a puncture-resistant sharps container located as close as possible to the area in which the items are used	☐ Yes ☐ No	
F. Sharps containers are disposed of in accordance with federal, state and local regulated medical waste rules and regulations	☐ Yes ☐ No	

II.5 Safe Injection Practices

Elements To Be Assessed	Assessment	Notes/Areas For Improvement
A. Injections are prepared using an aseptic technique in a clean area free from contaminants or contact with blood, body fluids, or contaminated equipment	☐ Yes ☐ No	
B. Needles and syringes are used for only one patient (this includes manufactured prefilled syringes and other devices such as insulin pens) **Note:** *When using a dental cartridge syringe to administer local anesthesia, do not use the needle, syringe, or anesthetic cartridge for more than one patient. Ensure that the dental cartridge syringe is appropriately cleaned and heat sterilized before use on another patient.*	☐ Yes ☐ No	
C. The rubber septum on a medication vial is disinfected with alcohol before piercing	☐ Yes ☐ No	
D. Medication containers (single and multidose vials, ampules, and bags) are entered with a new needle and a new syringe, even when obtaining additional doses for the same patient	☐ Yes ☐ No	
E. Single-dose (single-use) vials, ampules, and bags or bottles of intravenous solutions are used for only one patient	☐ Yes ☐ No	

continued on next page

II.5 Safe Injection Practices

Elements To Be Assessed	Assessment	Notes/Areas For Improvement
F. Leftover contents of single-dose vials, ampules, and bags of intravenous solutions are not combined for later use	☐ Yes ☐ No	
G. Single-dose vials for parenteral medications are used when possible	☐ Yes ☐ No	
H. When using multidose medication vials a. multidose vials are dedicated to individual patients whenever possible	☐ Yes ☐ No	
b. multidose vials to be used for more than one patient are kept in a centralized medication area and do not enter the immediate patient treatment area (e.g., dental operatory) to prevent inadvertent contamination of the vial **Note:** *If a multidose vial enters the immediate patient treatment area it should be dedicated for single-patient use and discarded immediately after use.*	☐ Yes ☐ No	
c. multidose vials are dated when first opened and discarded within 28 days unless the manufacturer specifies a shorter or longer date for that opened vial **Note:** *This is different from the expiration date printed on the vial.*	☐ Yes ☐ No	
I. Fluid infusion and administration sets (i.e., IV bags, tubings, and connections) are used for one patient only and disposed of appropriately	☐ Yes ☐ No	

II.6 Sterilization and Disinfection of Patient-Care Items and Devices

Elements To Be Assessed	Assessment	Notes/Areas For Improvement
A. Single-use devices are discarded after one use and not used for more than one patient	☐ Yes ☐ No	
B. Reusable critical and semicritical dental items and devices are cleaned and heat-sterilized according to manufacturer instructions between patient use **Note:** *If the manufacturer does not provide reprocessing instructions, the item or device may not be suitable for multi-patient use.*	☐ Yes ☐ No	
C. Items are thoroughly cleaned according to manufacturer instructions and visually inspected for residual contamination before sterilization	☐ Yes ☐ No	
D. Food and Drug Administration (FDA)-cleared automated cleaning equipment (e.g., ultrasonic cleaner, instrument washer, washer-disinfector) is used to remove debris to improve cleaning effectiveness and decrease worker exposure to blood	☐ Yes ☐ No	
E. Work-practice controls that minimize contact with sharp instruments (e.g., long-handled brush) are used and appropriate PPE is worn (e.g., punctureand chemical-resistant utility gloves) if manual cleaning is necessary	☐ Yes ☐ No	
F. After cleaning and drying, instruments are appropriately wrapped / packaged for sterilization (e.g., package system selected is compatible with the sterilization process being performed, hinged instruments are open, instruments are disassembled if indicated by the manufacturer)	☐ Yes ☐ No	

continued on next page

II.6 Sterilization and Disinfection of Patient-Care Items and Devices

Elements To Be Assessed	Assessment		Notes/Areas For Improvement
G. A chemical indicator is used inside each package. If the internal indicator is not visible from the outside, an exterior chemical indicator is also used on the package **Note:** *The chemical indicators may be integrated into the package design.*	☐ Yes	☐ No	
H. Sterile packs are labeled at a minimum with the sterilizer used, the cycle or load number, the date of sterilization, and if applicable an expiration date	☐ Yes	☐ No	
I. FDA-cleared medical devices for sterilization are used according to manufacturer's instructions	☐ Yes	☐ No	
J. A biologic indicator (i.e., spore test) is used at least weekly and with every load containing implantable items	☐ Yes	☐ No	
K. Logs for each sterilizer cycle are current and include results from each load and comply with state and local regulations	☐ Yes	☐ No	
L. After sterilization, dental devices and instruments are stored so that sterility is not compromised	☐ Yes	☐ No	
M. Sterile packages are inspected for integrity and compromised packages are reprocessed before use	☐ Yes	☐ No	
N. Instrument packs are not used if mechanical (e.g., time, temperature, pressure) or chemical indicators indicate inadequate processing (e.g., color change for chemical indicators)	☐ Yes	☐ No	
O. The instrument processing area has a workflow pattern designed to ensure that devices and instruments clearly flow from high contamination areas to clean / sterile areas (i.e., there is clear separation of contaminated and clean workspaces)	☐ Yes	☐ No	
P. Reusable heat sensitive semicritical items that cannot be replaced by a heat stable or disposable alternative are high-level disinfected according to manufacturer's instructions	☐ Yes	☐ No	
Q. High-level disinfection products are used and maintained according to manufacturer instructions	☐ Yes	☐ No	
R. Dental handpieces (including the low-speed motor) and other devices not permanently attachedto air and waterlines are cleaned and heat-sterilized according to manufacturer instructions	☐ Yes	☐ No	
S. If digital radiography is used in the dental setting — a. FDA-cleared barriers are used to cover the sensor and barriers are changed between patients b. after the surface barrier is removed, the sensor is ideally cleaned and heat sterilized or highlevel disinfected according to the manufacturer's instructions. If the item cannot tolerate these procedures, then at a minimum, the sensor is cleaned and disinfected with an intermediate level, EPA-registered hospital disinfectant	☐ Yes ☐ Yes	☐ No ☐ No	
Note: *Consult with manufacturers regarding compatibility of heat sterilization methods and disinfection products.*			

continued on facing page

II.7 Environmental Infection Prevention and Control

Elements To Be Assessed	Assessment	Notes/Areas For Improvement
A. Clinical contact surfaces are either barrier protected or cleaned and disinfected with an EPA-registered hospital disinfectant after each patient. An intermediate-level (i.e., tuberculocidal claim) disinfectant is used if visibly contaminated with blood	☐ Yes ☐ No	
B. Surface barriers are used to protect clinical contact surfaces that are difficult to clean (e.g., switches on dental chairs, computer equipment, connections to hoses) and are changed between patients	☐ Yes ☐ No	
C. Cleaners and disinfectants are used in accordance with manufacturer instructions (e.g., dilution, storage, shelf-life, contact time, PPE)	☐ Yes ☐ No	
D. Regulated medical waste is handled and disposed of according to local, state, and federal regulations	☐ Yes ☐ No	
E. DHCP engaged in environmental cleaning wear appropriate PPE to prevent exposure to infectious agents or chemicals (PPE can include gloves, gowns, masks, and eye protection) *Note:* The correct type of PPE depends on infectious or chemical agent and anticipated type of exposure.	☐ Yes ☐ No	

II.8 Dental Unit Water Quality

Elements To Be Assessed	Assessment	Notes/Areas For Improvement
A. Dental unit waterline treatment products / devices are used to ensure water meets EPA regulatory standards for drinking water (i.e., ≤ 500 CFU / mL of heterotrophic water bacteria) for routine dental treatment output water	☐ Yes ☐ No	
B. Product manufacturer instructions (i.e., waterline treatment product, dental unit manufacturer) are followed for monitoring the water quality	☐ Yes ☐ No	
C. Sterile saline or sterile water is used as a coolant / irrigant when performing surgical procedures *Note:* Use devices specifically designed for delivering sterile irrigating fluids (e.g., sterile bulb syringe, singleuse disposable products, and sterilizable tubing). *Note:* Examples of surgical procedures include biopsy, periodontal surgery, apical surgery, implant surgery, and surgical extractions of teeth.	☐ Yes ☐ No	

For more information please contact

Centers for Disease Control and Prevention

1600 Clifton Road NE, Atlanta, GA 30329-4027

Telephone: 1-800-CDC-INFO (232-4636)

TTY: 1-888-232-6348

E-mail: cdcinfo@cdc.gov

Web: www.cdc.gov/oralhealth

Publication Date: April 2016

Immunizing Agents And Immunization Schedules For Health-Care Personnel (HCP)*

Generic name	Primary schedule and booster(s)	Indications	Major precautions and contraindications	Special considerations
Immunizing agents recommended for all HCP				
Hepatitis B (HB) recombinant vaccine	2 doses 4 weeks apart; third dose 5 months after second; booster doses not necessary; all doses should be administered IM in the deltoid	Preexposure: HCP at risk for exposure to blood or body fluids; postexposure	On the basis of limited data, no risk for adverse effects to developing fetuses is apparent. Pregnancy should not be considered a contraindication to vaccination of women. Previous anaphylactic reaction to common baker's yeast is a contraindication to vaccination.	The vaccine produces neither therapeutic nor adverse effects in HBV-infected persons. Prevaccination serologic screening is not indicated for persons being vaccinated because of occupational risk but might be indicated for HCP in certain high-risk populations. HCP at high risk for occupational† contact with blood or body fluids should be tested 1–2 months after vaccination to determine serologic response.
Hepatitis B immune globulin (HBIG)	0.06 mL/kg IM as soon as possible after exposure, if indicated	Postexposure prophylaxis	See package insert§	
Influenza vaccine (TIV and LAIV)	Annual vaccination with current seasonal vaccine. TIV is available in IM and ID formulations. LAIV is administered intranasally.	All HCP	History of severe (e.g., anaphylactic) hypersensitivity to eggs; prior severe allergic reaction to influenza vaccine	No evidence exists of risk to mother of fetus when the vaccine is administered to a pregnant woman with an underlying high-risk condition. Influenza vaccination is recommended for women who are or will be pregnant during influenza season because of increased risk for hospitalization and death. LAIV is recommended only for healthy, non–pregnant persons aged 2–49 years. Intradermal vaccine is indicated for persons aged 18–64 years. HCP who care for severely immunosuppressed persons who require a protective environment should receive TIV rather than LAIV.
Measles live–virus vaccine	2 doses SC; ≥28 days apart	Vaccination should be recommended for all HCP who lack presumptive evidence of immunity;¶ vaccination should be considered for those born before 1957.	Pregnancy; immunocompromised persons,** including HIV-infected persons who have evidence of severe immunosuppression; anaphylaxis to gelatin or gelatin-containing products; anaphylaxis to neomycin; and recent administration of immune globulin.	HCP vaccinated during 1963–1967 with a killed measles vaccine alone, killed vaccine followed by live vaccine, or a vaccine of unknown type should be revaccinated with 2 doses of live measles virus vaccine.

See table footnotes on page 157

continued on facing page

From Policy to Practice: OSAP's Guide to the CDC Guidelines

Immunizing Agents and Immunization Schedules for Health-Care Personnel (HCP)*

continued from previous page

Generic name	Primary schedule and booster(s)	Indications	Major precautions and contraindications	Special considerations
Mumps live–virus vaccine	2 doses SC; ≥28 days apart	Vaccination should be recommended for all HCP who lack presumptive evidence of immunity.†† Vaccination should be considered for those born before 1957.	Pregnancy; immunocompromised persons,** including HIV-infected persons who have evidence of severe immunosuppression; anaphylaxis to gelatin or gelatin-containing products; anaphylaxis to	HCP vaccinated before 1979 with either killed mumps vaccine or mumps vaccine of unknown type should consider revaccination with 2 doses of MMR vaccine.
Rubella live-virus vaccine	1 dose SC; (However, due to the 2-dose requirements for measles and mumps vaccines, the use of MMR vaccine will result in most HCP receiving 2 doses of rubella-containing vaccine.)	Vaccination should be recommended for all HCP who lack presumptive evidence of immunity.§§	Pregnancy; immunocompromised persons** including HIV–infected persons who have evidence of severe immunosuppression; anaphylaxis to gelatin or gelatin–containing products; anaphylaxis to neomycin	The risk for rubella vaccine–associated malformations in the offspring of women pregnant when vaccinated or who become pregnant within 1 month after vaccination is negligible.¶¶ Such women should be counseled regarding the theoretical basis of concern for the fetus.
Tetanus and diphtheria (toxoids) and acellular pertussis (Tdap)	1 dose IM as soon as feasible if Tdap not already received and regardless of interval from last Td. After receipt of Tdap, receive Td for routine booster every 10 years.	All HCP, regardless of age.	History of serious allergic reaction (i.e., anaphylaxis) to any component of Tdap. Because of the importance of tetanus vaccination, persons with history of anaphylaxis to components in Tdap or Td should be referred to an allergist to determine whether they have a specific allergy to tetanus toxoid and can safely receive tetanus toxoid (TT) vaccine. Persons with history of encephalopathy (e.g., coma or prolonged seizures) not attributable to an identifiable cause within 7 days of administration of a vaccine with pertussis components should receive Td instead of Tdap.	Tetanus prophylaxis in wound management if not yet received Tdap***
Varicella vaccine (varicella zoster virus live-virus vaccine)	2 doses SC 4-6 weeks apart if aged ≥ 13 years.	All HCP who do not have evidence of immunity defined as: written documentation of vaccination with 2 doses of varicella vaccine: laboratory evidence of immunity††† or laboratory confirmation of disease; diagnosis or verification of a history of varicella disease by a health-care provider,§§§ or diagnosis or verification of a history of herpes zoster by a health-care provider.	Pregnancy; immunocompromised persons;** history of anaphylactic reaction after receipt of gelatin or neomycin. Varicella vaccination may be considered for HIV-infected adolescents and adults with CD4+ T-lymphocyte count >200 cells/uL. Avoid salicylate use for 6 weeks after vaccination.	Because 71%–93% of adults without a history of varicella are immune, serologic testing before vaccination is likely to be cost-effective.

See table footnotes on page 157

continued on next page

Immunizing Agents and Immunization Schedules for Health-Care Personnel (HCP)*

continued from previous page

Generic name	Primary schedule and booster(s)	Indications	Major precautions and contraindications	Special considerations
Varicella-zoster immune globulin	125U/10 kg IM (minimum dose: 125U; maximum dose: 625U)	Persons without evidence of immunity who have contraindications for varicella vaccination and who are at risk for severe disease and complications¶¶¶ known or likely to be susceptible who have direct, non-transient exposure to an infectious hospital staff worker or patient		Serologic testing may help in assessing whether to administer varicella–zoster immune globulin. If use of varicella–zoster immune globulin prevents varicella disease, patient should be vaccinated subsequently. The varicella–zoster immune globulin product currently used in the United States (VariZIG) (Cangene Corp. Winnipeg Canada) can be obtained 24 hours a day from the sole authorized U.S. distributor (FFF Enterprises, Temecula, California) at 1-800-843-7477 or www.fffenterprises.com.

Other immunobiologics that might be indicated in certain circumstances for HCP

Generic name	Primary schedule and booster(s)	Indications	Major precautions and contraindications	Special considerations
Quadrivalent meningococcal conjugate vaccine (tetravalent (A,C,Y,W) for HCP ages 19–54 years, Quadrivalent meningococcal polysaccharide vaccine for HCP age >55 years	1 dose; booster dose in 5 years if person remains at increased risk	Clinical and research microbiologists who might routinely be exposed to isolates of Neisseria meningitidis		The safety of the vaccine in pregnant women has not been evaluated; it should not be administered during pregnancy unless the risk for infection is high.
Typhoid vaccine IM, and oral	IM vaccine: 1 dose, booster every 2 years. Oral vaccine: 4 doses on alternate days. Manufacturer recommends revaccination with the entire 4-dose series every 5 years.	Workers in microbiology laboratories who frequently work with Salmonella typhi.	Severe local or systemic reaction to a previous dose. Ty21a (oral) vaccine should not be administered to immunocompromised persons** or to persons receiving antimicrobial agents.	Vaccination should not be considered an alternative to the use of proper procedures when handling specimens and cultures in the laboratory.
Inactivated poliovirus vaccine (IPV)	For unvaccinated adults, 2 doses should be administered at intervals of 4–8 weeks; a third dose should be administered 6–12 months after the second dose.	Vaccination is recommended for adults at increased risk for exposure to polioviruses including health-care personnel who have close contact with patients who might be excreting polioviruses. Adults who have previously received a complete course of poliovirus vaccine may receive one lifetime booster if they remain at increased risk for exposure.	Hypersensitivity or anaphylactic reactions to IPV or antibiotics contained in IPV. IPV contains trace amounts of streptomycin, polymyxin B, and neomycin.	

See table footnotes on page 157

Abbreviations:

IM	=	intramuscular;
HBV	=	hepatitis B virus;
HBsAg	=	hepatitis B surface antigen;
SC	=	subcutaneous;
HIV	=	human immunodeficiency virus;
MMR	=	measles, mumps, rubella vaccine;
TB	=	tuberculosis;
HAV	=	hepatitis A virus;
IgA	=	immune globulin A;
ID	=	intradermal;
TIV	=	trivalent inactivated split-virus vaccines;
LAIV	=	live attenuated influenza vaccine;
BCG	=	bacille Calmette-Guérin;
OPV	=	oral poliovirus vaccine.

* Persons who provide health care to patients or work in institutions that provide patient care (e. g., physicians, nurses, emergency medical personnel, dental professionals and students, medical and nursing students, laboratory technicians, hospital volunteers, and administrative and support staff in health-care institutions). Source: U.S. Department of Health and Human Services. Definition of health-care personnel (HCP). Available at : www.hhs.gov/ask/initiatives/vacctoolkit/definition.html.

† Health-care personnel and public safety workers at high risk for continued percutaneous or mucosal exposure to blood or body fluids include acupuncturists, dentists, dental hygienists, emergency medical technicians, first responders, laboratory technologists/technicians, nurses, nurse practitioners, phlebotomists, physicians, physician assistants, and students entering these professions. Source: CDC. A comprehensive immunization strategy to eliminate transmission of hepatitis B virus infection in the United States: recommendations of the Advisory Committee on Immunization Practices. Part II: immunization of adults. MMWR 2006;55(No. RR-16).

§ The package insert should be consulted to weigh the risks and benefits of giving HBIG to persons with IgA deficiency, or to persons who have had an anaphylactic reaction to an IgG containing biologic product.

¶ Written documentation of vaccination with 2 doses of live measles or MMR vaccine administered ≥28 days apart, or laboratory evidence of measles immunity, or laboratory confirmation of measles disease, or birth before 1957.

** Persons immunocompromised because of immune deficiency diseases, HIV infection (who should primarily not receive BCG, OPV, and yellow fever vaccines), leukemia, lymphoma or generalized malignancy or immunosuppressed as a result of therapy with corticosteroids, alkylating drugs, antimetabolites, or radiation.

†† Written documentation of vaccination with 2 doses of live mumps or MMR vaccine administered ≥28 days apart, or laboratory evidence of mumps immunity, or laboratory confirmation of mumps disease, or birth before 1957.

§§ Written documentation of vaccination with 1 dose of live rubella or MMR vaccine, or laboratory evidence of immunity, or laboratory confirmation of rubella infection or disease, or birth before 1957, except women of childbearing potential who could become pregnant; though pregnancy in this age group would be exceedingly rare.

¶¶ Source: CDC. Revised ACIP recommendation for avoiding pregnancy after receiving a rubella-containing vaccine. MMWR 2001;50:1117.

*** Source: CDC. Update on adult immunization: recommendations of the Advisory Committee on Immunization Practices (ACIP). MMWR 1991:40(No. RR-12).

††† Commercial assays can be used to assess disease–induced immunity, but they often lack sensitivity to detect vaccine-induced immunity (i.e., they might yield false-negative results).

§§§ Verification of history or diagnosis of typical disease can be provided by any health-care provider (e.g., school or occupational clinic nurse, nurse practitioner, physician assistant, or physician). For persons reporting a history of, or reporting with, atypical or mild cases, assessment by a physician or their designee is recommended, and one of the following should be sought: 1) an epidemiologic link to a typical varicella case or to a laboratory–confirmed case or 2) evidence of laboratory confirmation if it was performed at the time of acute disease. When such documentation is lacking, persons should not be considered as having a valid history of disease because other diseases might mimic mild atypical varicella.

¶¶¶ For example, immunocompromised patients or pregnant women.

Adapted from Centers for Disease Control and Prevention. Immunizations of Health-Care Personnel. Recommendations of the Advisory Committee on Immunization Practices (ACIP). MMWR Morbid Mortal Weekly Report November 25, 2011 / Vol. 60 / No. 7. Available at: www.cdc.gov/mmwr/pdf/rr/rr6007.pdf

Quick Reference Chart: Managing Patient-Care Items and Environmental Surfaces*

Process	Definition	Method		Examples	Used for ...	
Sterilization	Destroys all microorganisms, including bacterial spores	Heat automated	High temperature	Steam (autoclave), dry heat, unsaturated chemical vapor	Heat-tolerant critical and semicritical	
			Low temperature	Ethylene oxide gas, plasma sterilization	Heat-sensitive critical and semicritical	
		Liquid immersion§		Chemical sterilant (e.g., glutaraldehyde, glutaraldehyde with phenols, hydrogen peroxide, hydrogen peroxide with peracetic acid. peracetic acid)	Heat-sensitive critical and semicritical	
High-level disinfection	Destroys all microorganisms, but not necessarily high numbers of bacterial spores	Heat automated		Washer-disinfector	Heat-sensitive semicritical	
		Liquid immersion§		Chemical sterilant/high-level disinfectant (e.g., glutaraldehyde, orthophthalaldehyde, hydrogen peroxide, etc.)		
Intermediate-level disinfection	Destroys vegetative bacteria, most fungi, and most viruses; tuberculocidal; not necessarily capable of killing bacterial spores	Liquid contact — or — Barrier protection		Hospital disinfectant with label claim of tuberculocidal activity (e.g., chlorine-containing products, quaternary ammonium compounds with alcohol, phenolics, iodophors, EPA-registered chlorine-based products)	Noncritical with visible blood	Clinical contact surfaces
						Blood spills on housekeeping surfaces
Low-level disinfection	Destroys most vegetative bacteria, some fungi, and some viruses; not tuberculocidal	Liquid contact — or — Barrier protection		Hospital disinfectant with HBV and HIV claims but no tuberculocidal activity (e.g., quaternary ammonium compounds, some phenolics, some iodophors)	Noncritical without visible blood	Clinical contact surfaces that are thoroughly cleaned
						Housekeeping surfaces

* The U.S. Food and Drug Administration (FDA) regulates liquid sterilant/high-level disinfectants for use on critical and semicritical devices in healthcare settings. FDA also regulates medical devices, including sterilizers. Regulatory authority for intermediate- and low-level disinfectants for use on environmental surfaces falls to the U.S. Environmental Protection Agency (EPA).

§ Contact time is the single important variable distinguishing sterilization from high level disinfection with a liquid chemical sterilant/high-level disinfectant. The FDA defines a high-level disinfectant as a sterilant used under the same contact conditions as a steriliant except for a shorter immersion time (Food and Drug Administration 2000).

CDC Sample Device Screening and Evaluation Forms

The Centers for Disease Control and Prevention (CDC) has developed two sample forms (with instructions for use) to assist dental health care personnel in screening and evaluating the suitability of devices with engineered sharps safety features. Visit *www.cdc.gov/OralHealth/infectioncontrol/forms.htm* for more information.

Carefully read the introductions and instructions below to find out how to use the forms on pages 144 and 145 to assess the usefulness of sharps safety devices in your practice setting.

Developing Programs to Prevent Sharps Injuries

Your dental practice setting should develop and implement a program to prevent sharps injuries to dental health care personnel and patients. A staff person knowledgeable about or willing to be trained in injury prevention (a "safety coordinator") should be assigned to:

- promote safety awareness,
- facilitate prompt reporting and postexposure management of injuries,
- identify unsafe work practices and devices,
- coordinate the selection and evaluation of safer dental devices,
- organize staff education and training,
- complete the necessary reporting forms and documentation, and
- monitor safety performance.

These activities should be described in a written plan, and mechanisms for staff feedback should be available. This feedback will assist your safety coordinator in monitoring the effectiveness of the plan and making modifications if needed.

Identifying and Setting Priorities for Safer Dental Devices

Get information on specific brands and types of safer dental devices from vendors, purchasing agents, the scientific literature, lists published on the Internet or in trade journals, and other dental facilities. Consider a variety of devices; don't limit your choices to products available from any one vendor.

Evaluating sharps safety devices is a two-step process ("screening" and "device evaluation"). Each step requires its own set of predetermined evaluation criteria that will help to objectively assess the usefulness of each safety device in preventing injuries within your practice setting. Criteria used in both phases of the assessment should be easy to understand, and the forms used to record dental health care personnel opinions should be easy to read and score.

Screening Devices

The first step — screening — helps dental health care personnel make decisions about clinical and safety considerations before bringing a safety device into the patient-care setting. Screening usually consists of physically examining the safety device, then comparing it to the traditional device and the evaluation criteria your practice setting has decided are important. The goal of screening is to determine whether a device is safe for use on patients, if it has a safety feature that could protect dental health care personnel from sharps injury, and if it is readily available for purchase, easy and practical to use, and compatible with other equipment.

Never use a sharps safety device on a patient before it has been screened to make sure that it meets clinical and patient-safety needs.

Evaluating Devices

The second step — device evaluation — involves a trial (a "pilot test") to examine the device's performance under clinical circumstances in your practice setting. It includes identifying a safer dental device to test, selecting the area of the facility in which it will be used, identifying the workers who will test the device, selecting evaluation criteria, determining how long the test will last, and plans for quickly bringing back the traditional device if the test device is found to be less safe.

Only devices that have "passed" the screening phase should be tested during patient care. Criteria for the device evaluation phase help determine a safety device's impact on patient care, user acceptability, and cost. Device evaluation should provide your safety coordinator with enough information to make an informed decision on whether to make the safety device a permanent part of your practice setting's injury prevention program.

Sample Forms

Although the CDC designed its sample forms so they are specific for anesthetic syringes, the forms can be modified for use with other types of dental devices and to include any additional evaluation criteria required in your specific practice setting.

CDC Sample Screening Form

Instructions for Using the Sample Screening Form

Adapting the Form. The form can be modified to address your specific clinical needs by adding criteria that reflect the situation in your practice setting or deleting criteria that are not appropriate. For example, if your patient population consists primarily of children, you may choose to add criteria that reflect the use of the device in small mouths.

Obtaining Feedback. In the screening phase, include a representative of each type of dental health care personnel that will be using or handling the device. Each person completing a form should have a sample of the safer device as well as the traditional device in front of them.

Interpreting the Results. Once the form has been completed by everyone involved in the screening process, discuss the results to determine whether to proceed to the next phase – evaluating the safer device in the clinical setting. In making this decision, some criteria may be more important than others. For example, clinical and safety feature considerations may be more important than the general-product or practical considerations. If the responses to many criteria are "Does Not Meet Expectations" or "No," then you should consider other safer devices; otherwise, evaluate the device in the clinical setting.

Sample Screening Form for Dental Safety Syringes and Needles

This form collects the opinions and observations of dental health care personnel who screen a safer dental device to determine its acceptability for use in a clinical setting. This form can be adapted for use with multiple types of devices. Do not use the test safety device on a patient during this initial screening phase.

Date:_____   Product Name, Brand, Company: _____

Your position or title: _____   Your occupation or specialty: _____

Respond to each statement with either: (a) "Yes" or "No," or

(b) a numerical rating   **1 = Exceeds Expectations   2 = Meets Expectations   3 = Does Not Meet Expectations**

Clinical Considerations

1. The device permits the exchange of cartridges during treatment on the same patient.   1   2   3
2. The weight and size of the device is acceptable.   1   2   3
3. I have a clear view of the cartridge contents when aspirating.   1   2   3
4. The size and configuration of the syringe or needle permits a clear view of the injection site and needle tip.   1   2   3
5. No excessive force is required to activate or control the plunger.   1   2   3
6. The size and configuration of the syringe or needle permits use in all mouth sizes and access to all areas of the mouth.   1   2   3
7. The device permits multiple injections on the same patient.   Yes   No
8. The device is capable of aspiration before injection.   Yes   No
9. The needle is compatible with a reusable syringe. [For safety needles without syringes only.]   Yes   No

   Does the product meet the needs of your clinical practice based on the above criteria?   Yes   No
10. The worker's hands can remain behind the sharp during activation of the safety feature.   1   2   3

Safety Feature Considerations

11. The safety feature can be activated with one hand.   1   2   3
12. The safety feature is integrated into the syringe or needle.   1   2   3
13. The safety feature provides a temporary means of protecting the needle between injections.   1   2   3
14. A visible or audible cue provides evidence of safety feature activation.   1   2   3

15. The safety feature is easy to recognize and use.   Yes   No
16. Once activated, the safety feature permanently isolates the needle tip and cannot be purposefully or accidentally deactivated under normal use conditions.   Yes   No
17. The safety feature activates by itself.   Yes   No

General Product/Manufacturer Considerations

18. Manufacturer can provide the device in needed quantities.   1   2   3
19. A full range of needle sizes and lengths is available.   1   2   3
20. The company provides free samples for in-use evaluation.   1   2   3
21. The company has a history of responsiveness to problems.   1   2   3

Practical Considerations

22. The device is packaged conveniently.   1   2   3
23. The device is easy to remove aseptically from the package.   1   2   3
24. Instructions are included in the packaging.   1   2   3
25. Instructions are easy to follow and complete.   1   2   3
26. Instructions are provided in more than one form (paper, videotape, website, or computer disk).   1   2   3
27. Use of the safety device will not increase the volume of sharps waste.   1   2   3
28. The shape and size of available sharps containers will accommodate disposal of this device.   1   2   3
29. This is a single use, disposable device.   Yes   No
30. The device should be considered for further clinical evaluation.   Yes   No

Additional comments for any responses of "Does Not Meet Expectations" or "No."

_____

_____

CDC Sample Device Evaluation Form

Instructions for Using the Sample Device Evaluation Form

Adapting the Form. Like the screening form, the device evaluation form can be modified to address your clinical needs by adding criteria that reflect the situation in your practice setting or by deleting criteria that are less relevant.

Obtaining Feedback. Select staff who represent the scope of workers who will use or handle the device. Choose a reasonable testing period (2 to 4 weeks should be sufficient). Staff should receive training on correct use of the device, which often can be provided by product representatives. Staff are encouraged to provide informal feedback during the evaluation period. Your safety coordinator should monitor this pilot test to ensure proper use of the safer device and remove the device immediately if it is found to be unsafe. Complete and return forms to the safety coordinator as soon as possible after the evaluation period.

Interpreting the Results. After the evaluation phase, your safety coordinator should speak with workers who have completed the forms to determine the criteria that should receive the most consideration. For example, workers may express that criteria regarding the "feel" of the device (for example, its weight and size, how it fits in their hand) are important in maintaining proper injection technique. If the responses to many of the criteria are "Strongly Disagree" or "Disagree," workers who have completed the form should be asked to provide additional information. This feedback should be balanced with safety and practical considerations before determining whether to continue using the device in your practice.

Sample Screening Form for Dental Safety Syringes and Needles

This form collects opinions and observations from dental health care personnel who have pilot-tested a safer dental device. This form can be adapted for use with multiple types of safer devices. **Do not use this form to collect injury data because it cannot ensure confidentiality.**

Date:_____   Product Name, Brand, Company: _____   No. of Times You Used the Device: _____

Your position or title: _____   Your occupation or specialty: _____

1. Did you receive training in how to use this product?   ❏ Yes [Go to Next Question]   ❏ No [Go to Question 4]

2. Who provided this instruction? (Check all that apply.)   ❏ Product representative   ❏ Staff member   ❏ Other

3. Was the training you received adequate?   ❏ Yes   ❏ No

4. Compared to others of your sex, how would you describe your hand size?   ❏ Small   ❏ Medium   ❏ Large

5. What is your sex?   ❏ Female   ❏ Male

Respond to each statement: **1 = Strongly Agree**   **2 = Agree**   **3 = Neither Agree nor Disagree**   **4 = Disagree**   **5 = Strongly Disagree**

6. The weight of the device was similar to that of a conventional dental syringe.	1 2 3 4 5	15. I used the device for all of the same purposes for which I used the conventional device.	1 2 3 4 5
7. The device felt stable during assembly, use and disassembly.	1 2 3 4 5	16. Activating the safety feature was easy.	1 2 3 4 5
8. The device fit my hand comfortably.	1 2 3 4 5	17. The safety feature was easy to recognize and use.	1 2 3 4 5
9. The anesthetic cartridges were easy to change.	1 2 3 4 5	18. The safety feature did not activate inadvertently, causing me to use additional syringes or needles.	1 2 3 4 5
10. Aspiration of blood into the anesthetic cartridge was clearly visible.	1 2 3 4 5	19. The safety feature functioned as intended.	1 2 3 4 5
11. I had a clear view of the injection site and needle tip.	1 2 3 4 5	20. The instructions were easy to follow and complete.	1 2 3 4 5
12. The device did not appear to increase patient discomfort.	1 2 3 4 5	21. I could have used this product correctly without special training.	1 2 3 4 5
13. The device performed reliably.	1 2 3 4 5	22. The "feel" of the device did not cause me to change my technique.	1 2 3 4 5
14. I was able to give injections in all mouth sizes and all areas of the mouth.	1 2 3 4 5	23. This device meets my clinical needs.	1 2 3 4 5
		24. This device is safe for clinical use.	1 2 3 4 5

Additional comments for any responses of "Does Not Meet Expectations" or "No."

_____

_____

_____

_____

Selected Resources for Infection Control Compliance and Product Information

Agencies and Associations

American Dental Association
Infection control recommendations, position statements, literature, and information
www.ada.org/en/member-center/oral-health-topics/infection-control-resources

American Public Health Association
Group of public health professionals (researchers, health service providers, administrators, teachers, and health workers) focusing on personal and environmental health
apha.org/

Association for Professionals in Infection Control and Epidemiology, Inc.
Nonprofit, international organization dedicated to communicating information to persons involved in infection control
www.apic.org/

Centers for Disease Control and Prevention, Div. of Oral Health
Dental infection control fact sheets, frequently asked questions and answers, guidelines, publications, and more
www.cdc.gov/OralHealth/infectioncontrol/index.htm

Centers for Disease Control and Prevention, Div. of Healthcare Quality Promotion
Infection control guidelines, information, and publications for healthcare workers
www.cdc.gov/ncezid/dhqp/index.html

Centers for Disease Control and Prevention, National Prevention Information Network
Information and resources on HIV/AIDS, STD, and TB prevention
npin.cdc.gov/

Dental Assistant National Board, Inc.
National certification board for dental assistants.
www.danb.org

HIVdent.org
Information on providing oral health services to the HIV-infected population
www.hivdent.org

OSAP-DANB-Dale Foundation Collaboration
Dental infection control education program and two professional certifications
dentalinfectioncontrol.org

National Institute for Occupational Health and Safety
Resources for identifying and guarding against workplace hazards
www.cdc.gov/niosh/

Occupational Safety and Health Administration
Regulatory information specific to dental settings
www.osha.gov/SLTC/dentistry/index.html

Bloodborne Pathogens Standard resources and compliance information
www.osha.gov/SLTC/bloodbornepathogens/index.html

State OSHA Plans
www.osha.gov/dcsp/osp/

OSAP / Organization for Safety, Asepsis and Prevention.
In-depth look at current infection control issues of interest to DHCP. Guidelines, position papers, frequently asked questions and answers, and more
www.osap.org

State and Local Health Departments
Directory of links
www.cdc.gov/mmwr/international/relres.html

Postexposure Management

Emergency Needlestick Information
Centers for Disease Control and Prevention
www.cdc.gov/niosh/topics/bbp/emergnedl.html

Clinicians' Post Exposure Prophylaxis (PEP) Line:
1-888-488-4911
nccc.ucsf.edu/clinician-consultation/pep-post-exposure-prophylaxis/

Employer Obligations After Exposure Incidents OSHA
www.ada.org/en/science-research/osha-standard-of-occupational-exposure-to-bloodbor

Product Information

American Association for the Advancement of Medical Instrumentation
Voluntary standards for sterilization equipment and biological monitoring manufacturers in the U.S.
www.aami.org/

American Dental Association
Seal of Acceptance Program
www.ada.org/en/public-programs/ ada-seal-of-acceptance-program/

ADA Standards Committee on Dental Products (SCDP) and its work on American National Standards for dental products
www.ada.org/en/science-research/ dental-standards/

American National Standards Institute
Voluntary standards for products produced in the U.S.
ansi.org/

Centers for Disease Control and Prevention, Div. of Oral Health
Instructions and sample forms for evaluating safer sharps devices within the dental practice setting
www.cdc.gov/OralHealth/

Dental Products Report
Online and print trade journal highlighting new dental products and featuring a monthly infection control article
www.dentalproductsreport.com/

Dentistry Today
Online and print trade journal highlighting new dental products
www.dentistrytoday.com/

Environmental Protection Agency
Listings of EPA's registered antimicrobial products
www.epa.gov/pesticide-registration/select-ed-epa-registered-disinfectants

Food and Drug Administration, Center for Devices and Radiological Health
Regulatory information and medical device databases
www.fda.gov/AboutFDA/CentersOffices/Offic eofMedicalProductsandTobacco/CDRH/ default.htm
Searchable database containing a listing of medical devices in commercial distribution by both domestic and foreign manufacturers
www.fda.gov/medicaldevices/device regulationandguidance/databases/default.htm

510(k) database
www.fda.gov/MedicalDevices/ProductsandM edicalProcedures/DeviceApprovalsand Clearances/510kClearances/ucm089319.htm

MEDWATCH medical device adverse events reporting
www.fda.gov/Safety/MedWatch/

National Institute for Occupational Health and Safety
Selecting, Evaluating, and Using Sharps Disposal Containers
www.cdc.gov/niosh/docs/97-111/

Training for Development of Innovative Control Technologies Project
Injury prevention tools and performance standards

Publications: Regulatory, Research, and Professional Interest

ADHA Publications
Magazine of the American Dental Hygienists' Association
adha.org/ publications/index.html

AEGIS Communications
Publishes Inside Dentistry, the Compendium of Continuing Education in Dentistry, Inside Dental Technology and CDEWorld.
www.dentalaegis.com/about

Dental Assistant Journal
Journal of the American Dental Assistants Association
www.adaausa.org/Publications/ Dental-Assistant-Journa

Federal Register
Official daily publication for rules, proposed rules, and notices of U.S. agencies and organizations
www.gpoaccess.gov/fr/ index.html

GPO / Government Printing Office
Searchable database containing the *Federal Register*, Congressional Reports, laws, and Supreme Court decisions
www.gpoaccess.gov/multidb.html

Infection Control Today
Journal focusing on infection control in health care
www.infectioncontroltoday.com/

Infection Control and Hospital Epidemiology Journal
journals.cambridge.org/action/ displayJournal?jid=ICE

Morbidity and Mortality Weekly Report
Published by the Centers for Disease Control and Prevention
www.cdc.gov/mmwr/index.html

Journal of Dental Infection Control and Safety
This is the official journal of OSAP focusing on dental infection control and safety
osapjdics.scholasticahq.com/

Infection Control In Practice
Official OSAP newsletter focusing on one infection control and safety topic of interest per issue
www.OSAP.org

Pennwell Publishing
Publishers of *Dental Equipment and Materials*, *Dental Economics*, and *RDH*
www.pennwell.com/industries/ dental.html

PubMed
The National Library of Medicine's searchable database
www.ncbi.nlm.nih.gov/PubMed

Glossary of Terms You Should Know

— A —

Administrative controls The use of administrative measures (that is, policies and procedures) to reduce the risk of exposure to pathogenic organisms.

Aerosols Particles of a size that can be inhaled (less than 10 microns) generated by both humans and environmental sources that can survive and remain airborne for extended periods in the indoor environment. Sources of aerosols in the dental setting include the use of handpieces, ultrasonic scalers, and air-water syringes.

AIDS Acquired Immune Deficiency Syndrome, which is caused by infection with the human immunodeficiency virus (HIV) and is characterized by a weakening of the immune system.

Airborne transmission A means of spreading infection in which microscopic airborne particles (droplet nuclei) are inhaled by the susceptible host. Also see *Droplet nuclei.*

Alcohol-based hand rub An alcohol-containing waterless antiseptic preparation that is rubbed onto the hands without wetting or rinsing to reduce the number of microorganisms on the skin.

Allergen A substance capable of inducing allergy or specific hypersensitivity.

Allergic contact dermatitis A skin reaction resulting from contact with a chemical allergen (for example, poison ivy, certain components of patient-care gloves, some dental materials), generally confined to the contact area and appearing slowly over 12-48 hours. Also referred to as "type IV" or "delayed" hypersensitivity.

Anaphylaxis A sudden, severe, potentially fatal systemic allergic reaction with symptoms that can include hives, watery eyes, and difficulty breathing. Also referred to as "type I" or "immediate" hypersensitivity.

Antibody A protein produced by the immune system in response to the presence of a specific antigen (that is, a foreign body/agent such as a virus); it helps the body fight infection.

Antimicrobial agent A product that has the ability to kill or otherwise irreversibly destroy microorganisms.

Antiseptic A germicide used on skin or living tissue to inhibit or kill microorganisms; examples include alcohols, chlorhexidine, chlorine, hexachlorophene, iodine, chloroxylenol (PCMX), quaternary ammonium compounds, and triclosan.

Antiseptic handwash Washing hands with water and a soap/detergent that contains an antiseptic agent.

Antiseptic hand rub Applying an alcohol-based hand-rub product to all surfaces of the hands to reduce the number of microorganisms present.

Appliance A fixed or removable corrective dental device that replaces, holds, or moves teeth, for example, partial denture, orthodontic retainer.

Asepsis The absence of contamination.

Aseptic technique Manner of safe handling and use that prevents or reduces the spread of microorganisms from one site to another.

— B —

Bacterial count Method of estimating the number of bacteria per unit sample; also refers to the estimated number of bacteria per unit sample, often expressed as colony-forming units per milliliter (CFU/mL).

Bacterial endocarditis An infection of the heart's inner lining (endocardium) or the heart valves; occurs when bacteria in the bloodstream lodge on abnormal heart valves or other damaged heart tissue.

Barrier An item that blocks the penetration of microorganisms, particulates, and fluids, thereby reducing the potential contamination of the underlying surface. Also referred to as "surface barrier."

Bioburden (1) Organic material on a surface or object prior to cleaning or sterilization; (2) the number of viable organisms in or on the object or surface. Also known as "bioload" or "microbial load."

Biological indicator Device that monitors the sterilization process by using a standardized population of resistant bacterial spores; verifies that all the parameters necessary for sterilization were present. Also called "spore test" or "BI."

Biofilm An assemblage of microbial cells that is irreversibly associated (not removed by gentle rinsing) with a surface and enclosed in a matrix of primarily polysaccharide material.

Biohazard A biological agent (such as an infectious microorganism) or a condition that poses a threat to humans.

Biohazard symbol Universal indicator of an infectious hazard; indicated by the symbol " ."

Biopsy Removal and examination of tissue, cells, or fluid from a living patient.

Bloodborne disease An illness that is transmitted by exposure to pathogens in the blood.

Bloodborne pathogen A disease-producing microorganism spread by contact with blood or other body fluids contaminated with blood from an infected person; examples include hepatitis B virus, hepatitis C virus, and HIV.

— C —

Carrier A person, immune or recovered from a disease, who still harbors and can transmit the infectious agent to others.

CFU/mL See *Colony-forming units per milliliter.*

Chain of Infection The set of five conditions — all of which must be present — that allows disease transmission to occur; includes (1) a pathogen in sufficient numbers to cause infection, (2) a place for the pathogen to reside and multiply; (3) a mode of transmission to transfer the pathogen to the new host; (4) a portal of entry into a new host (that is, an appropriate route for the pathogen to enter the body); and (5) a host that is not immune to the pathogen. Infection control efforts remove one or more "links" in the chain of infection, thereby preventing disease transmission.

Chemical indicator Device that monitors the sterilization process by changing color or form with exposure to one or more sterilizing conditions (for example, temperature, steam); intended to detect potential sterilization failures due to incorrect packaging, incorrect sterilizer loading, or equipment malfunction.

Cleaning Removing visible contamination from a device or surface, using either the physical action of scrubbing with a surfactant/detergent and water or an energy-based process (such as that used by an ultrasonic cleaner) with the appropriate chemical agents.

Clinical contact surface Surfaces that are touched by contaminated hands, instruments, devices, or other items while providing dental or medical care or while performing activities that support dental or medical care.

Colonize To establish a mass of microorganisms in or on a solid surface.

Colony-forming units per milliliter The minimum number (that is, tens of millions) of separable cells that gives rise to visible growth; may consist of pairs, chains, and clusters as well as single cells. Abbreviated "CFU/mL."

Confidentiality The safeguarding of information, protection of private or sensitive information.

Conscious sedation Anesthesia: A minimally depressed level of consciousness in which the patient retains the ability to independently and continuously maintain an airway and respond appropriately to physical stimulation, verbal command, and/or pain.

Contact time The exposure time for a disinfectant to accomplish the desired antimicrobial effect, as defined by the disinfectant manufacturer.

Contaminated / Contamination The presence of microorganisms (usually those capable of producing disease or infection) on living or nonliving surfaces.

Critical The category of medical devices or instruments that cut or otherwise penetrate bone or soft tissue, providing them with access to the bloodstream or normally unexposed tissues; so named because of the substantial risk of acquiring infection if such an item is contaminated.

Cross-contamination Spreading microorganisms between persons and/or surfaces.

Culture of safety A prevention strategy based on the shared commitment of everyone in a facility toward ensuring the safety of the work environment, the dental personnel, and the patients.

— D —

Decontamination Process or treatment that makes a medical device, instrument, or environmental surface safe (that is, no longer capable of transmitting a disease) to handle, use, or discard.

Delayed hypersensitivity See *Allergic contact dermatitis.*

Dental treatment water Nonsterile water used during dental treatment, such as for irrigating nonsurgical operative sites and cooling highspeed rotary and ultrasonic instruments.

Detergent Compound with cleaning action but no antimicrobial activity; also referred to as "soap."

Direct contact Physical transfer of microorganisms between an infected or colonized person and a susceptible host.

Disinfectant Chemical agent used on inanimate (nonliving) objects to destroy virtually all recognized pathogens, but not necessarily bacterial endospores.

Disinfection Destruction of pathogenic and other kinds of microorganisms by physical or chemical means; less lethal than sterilization, it destroys most recognized pathogens but does not necessarily kill bacterial spores. See *High-level disinfection, Intermediate-level disinfection,* and *Low-level disinfection.*

Disposable See *Single-use.*

Droplet nuclei Potentially infectious microscopic particles (5 microns or less in diameter) that can remain suspended in the air for long periods of time; formed by the dehydration of airborne droplets containing microorganisms. Also see *Airborne transmission.*

Droplets / spatter Small particles of moisture expelled into the air, as when a person coughs or sneezes or when water is converted to a fine mist by an aerator or shower head. Larger than droplet nuclei, these particles may contain infectious microorganisms but quickly settle on surfaces, usually limiting the risk of disease transmission to persons near the source of the droplets.

Engineering controls Controls that isolate or remove the bloodborne pathogens hazard from a workplace; examples include sharps disposal containers and safer medical devices (such as self-sheathing needles and needleless systems).

Environmental Protection Agency Bureau of the United States government charged with regulating disinfectants used on environmental surfaces (intermediate- and low-level disinfectants) and waste generated in healthcare facilities. Abbreviated "EPA."

Environmental controls Tuberculosis transmission: Series of precautions aimed at limiting the spread of a pathogen via the surrounding air; includes negatively pressured isolation rooms, ventilation to outside air, and systems to filter microscopic particles from the air.

Environmental surface Surface within a dental or medical treatment area that is not directly involved in patient care that may or may not be contaminated during the course of treatment; examples include countertops, drawer handles, floors, walls, and instrument control panels. Also see *Clinical contact surface* and *Housekeeping surface*.

EPA See *Environmental Protection Agency*.

EPA Registration number A hyphenated two- or three-part number assigned by the Environmental Protection Agency to identify each germicidal product registered within the United States. Indicated by "EPA Reg. No." on a product's label.

Event-related packaging A storage practice that recognizes that a package and its contents should remain sterile until some event causes the item(s) to become contaminated.

Expiration date Date past which a product should not be used.

Exposure control plan A healthcare facility's written protocols for reducing the risk of occupational exposures.

Exposure incident A specific eye, mouth, other mucous membrane, non-intact skin, or parenteral contact with blood or other potentially infectious materials that results from the performance of a worker's duties.

Exposure prevention Series of steps to minimize or eliminate dental health care personnels' risks of acquiring a disease in the course of their work; includes administrative controls, engineering controls, personal protective equipment, work practice controls, handwashing, and immunizations.

Exposure management Series of steps carried out in the event of an accidental exposure; includes first aid, immediate reporting, and referral to a qualified healthcare professional for evaluation and follow-up.

Exposure time Period of time during a sterilization or disinfection process in which items are exposed to a sterilant or disinfectant at the parameters specified by the manufacturer (for example, time, concentration, temperature, pressure).

Face shield Personal protective equipment: A solid, clear plastic barrier that covers the eyes and possibly the nose and mouth to protect against splash and spatter.

FDA See *Food and Drug Administration*.

Filter Dental waterlines: A device placed within the waterline to trap microscopic organisms in the water before they are delivered to the patient or the environment.

Fluid infusion system System for delivering intravenous fluids to patients; includes IV bags, flowmeter, tubing, and an intravenous catheter.

Flushing The act of running water through waterlines and/or the devices attached to them.

Food and Drug Administration Bureau of the United States government that regulates medical devices such as sterilizers, instrument cleaners, gloves, syringes, surgical masks, and dental alloys. Abbreviated "FDA."

Germicide An agent that destroys microorganisms, especially pathogenic organisms. Other terms with the suffix "–cide" (for example, virucide, fungicide, bactericide, tuberculocide, sporicide) use the prefix to indicate the type of microorganisms that are inactivated (for example, a virucide inactivates viruses). Antiseptics are germicides for living tissue; disinfectants are germicides used on nonliving items and surfaces.

Gloves Personal protective equipment: Barriers that protect the hands against contamination.

— H —

Hand antisepsis General term that describes *Antiseptic handwash* and *Antiseptic hand rub*.

Hand hygiene General term that describes *Handwashing*, *Antiseptic handwash*, *Antiseptic hand rub*, and *Surgical hand antisepsis*.

Handpiece A rotary cutting instrument powered by compressed air or electric motors; used to prepare cavities for fillings, adjust bites, etc.

Handwashing Using a plain or antimicrobial soap-and-water lather followed by a water rinse to remove debris from hands.

HBIG See *Hepatitis B immune globulin*.

HBV See *Hepatitis B virus*.

HCV See *Hepatitis C virus*.

Healthcare-associated infection Any infection associated with a medical or surgical intervention.

Heat sterilization A heat process that destroys all microbial life, including bacterial endospores. Autoclaves, chemical-vapor sterilizers, and dry-heat sterilizers are used in dentistry for heat sterilization of patient-care items.

Hepatitis An inflammation of the liver that can be caused by viruses, bacteria, trauma, drug reactions, or alcoholism.

Hepatitis B immune globulin A product prepared from plasma containing high titers of hepatitis B antibodies that provides short-term protection (3-6 mos.) against hepatitis B infection; may be used in postexposure prophylaxis. Abbreviated "HBIG."

Hepatitis B virus A highly transmissible bloodborne disease agent that can cause a form of liver damage; a serious occupational risk to unvaccinated DHCP. Abbreviated "HBV."

Hepatitis C virus A bloodborne disease agent that can result in very serious liver disease. Abbreviated "HCV."

High-level disinfectant U.S. Food and Drug Administration term describing a liquid chemical sterilant used for a shorter contact time; inactivates vegetative bacteria, mycobacteria, fungi, and viruses but not necessarily high numbers of bacterial spores.

High-level disinfection A process that inactivates vegetative bacteria, mycobacteria, fungi, and viruses but not necessarily high numbers of bacterial spores. See *High-level disinfectant*.

HIV The human immunodeficiency virus; HIV infection may develop into AIDS.

Hospital disinfectant A germicide registered by the U.S. Environmental Protection Agency that is effective against the test microorganisms *Salmonella choleraesuis*, *Staphylococcus aureus*, and *Pseudomonas aeruginosa* for use on nonliving objects in dental and medical facilities.

Host Person, animal, or plant on which or in which a foreign microorganism lives.

Housekeeping surface Environmental surface that is not involved in the direct delivery of dental care (for example, floors, walls).

— I —

Immediate hypersensitivity see *Anaphylaxis*.

Immunity Protection against a disease; indicated by the presence of antibodies in the blood, which usually can be identified with a laboratory test.

Immunocompetent Having a healthy immune response.

Immunocompromised Having an immune system that cannot adequately respond to challenges.

Immunization The process by which a person becomes immune, or protected, against a disease. Also see *Vaccination* and *Vaccine*.

Implantable device A device that is placed into a surgically or naturally formed cavity of the human body where it is meant to remain for at least 30 days.

Impression A mold, or negative, of a tooth or teeth that is used to make crowns, bridges, veneers, dentures, space maintainers, and some fillings.

Independent water reservoir See *Self-contained water system*.

Indirect contact Contact between a susceptible host and a contaminated object that is not the original source of the contamination (for example, instruments, equipment, or environmental surfaces).

Infection Control Coordinator Person within a dental practice setting responsible for establishing infection control policies and standard operating procedures, managing exposure incidents, coordinating infection control training and record-keeping, and ensuring compliance with all applicable regulations and recommendations.

Intermediate-level disinfection Disinfection process that inactivates vegetative bacteria, most fungi, mycobacteria, and most viruses but not bacterial spores.

Intermediate-level disinfectant A liquid chemical germicide registered with the U.S. Environmental Protection Agency as a hospital disinfectant with tuberculocidal activity.

Invasive procedure An examination or treatment that penetrates tissue or otherwise causes bleeding.

Irritant contact dermatitis Dry, itchy, irritated areas of the skin caused by physical irritation (such as friction or dehydration), not an allergic reaction; may result from frequent handwashing and gloving as well as exposure to chemicals.

IV catheter A medical device inserted into a vein to deliver fluids.

— L —

Latex hypersensitivity A potentially serious allergic reaction to the proteins found in natural rubber latex; also called a "type I" or "immediate" hypersensitivity.

Local Health care: Involving or affecting only a limited part of the body; for example, a "local anesthetic," or a "local infection."

Low-level disinfectant A hospital disinfectant that may also have a label claim for effectiveness against hepatitis B virus and HIV. See *Hospital disinfectant*.

Low-level disinfection Process that inactivates most vegetative bacteria, some fungi, and some viruses but cannot be relied on to inactivate resistant microorganisms (for example, mycobacteria or bacterial spores).

— M —

Malaise A generalized feeling of discomfort, illness, or lack of well being that can be associated with a disease state.

Mask Personal protective equipment: Surgical mask: A barrier for the face that covers the nose and mouth to protect against splash and spatter.

Mechanical indicator Device (such as a gauge, meter, display, or printout) that displays an element of the sterilization process (for example, time, temperature, pressure).

Medical gloves Barriers that protect the hands against contamination during patient care; supplied either nonsterile or sterile.

Medical records In the context of this workbook, dental DHCP occupational health records that must be maintained and kept confidential by the employer or a designated healthcare professional; may only include hepatitis B vaccination information, any exposure incident reports, and written confirmation of postexposure evaluation from a qualified healthcare professional.

Medical waste Waste generated through the provision of medical or dental care; may be regulated or nonregulated.

Mercury A heavy, silver-white metallic element bound into the alloys used as dental amalgam; hazardous when vaporized under high temperatures.

Microfilter Membrane filter with a pore size of 0.03-10 microns that traps microorganisms suspended in water; often installed on dental unit waterlines near the point of use as a retrofit device; different from large-pore (20-90 micron) sediment filters commonly found in dental unit water regulators, which do not function as microbiological filters.

Microorganism An organism of microscopic or ultramicroscopic size; includes bacteria, viruses, fungi, endospores, mycobacteria.

Mode of transmission The means by which pathogens are transferred to a new host. See *Chain of infection.*

Mouthrinse A preparation for cleansing the mouth and teeth; may contain fluoride, antiseptic, or odor inhibitors. Also see *Preprocedural mouthrinse.*

Mucous membranes Soft tissue that lines body passages and cavities (for example, the eyes, mouth, and nose), secreting fluids that moisten and protect the area.

— N —

N-95 respirator Type of disposable, air-purifying respirator that filters 95% of microscopic particles from the air; approved by the National Institute for Occupational Safety and Health (NIOSH) as personal protective equipment to prevent tuberculosis exposure. Must be tested prior to use to ensure that it fits well enough to be effective.

Natural rubber latex A milky white fluid extracted from the rubber tree *Hevea brasiliensis*; found in some gloves, orthodontic bands, anesthesia masks, goggles, and other household and medical devices.

Noncritical Instruments or surfaces that contact only intact skin.

Nosocomial infection An infection acquired in a hospital as a result of medical care.

— O —

Occupational exposure Any reasonably anticipated skin, eye, mucous membrane, or percutaneous contact with blood or other potentially infectious materials that may result from the performance of an employee's duties.

Occupational injury An acute exposure, such as a cut, splash, scrape, or puncture wound, sustained during the course of performing job responsibilities and requiring immediate reporting, evaluation by a qualified healthcare professional, and if necessary, follow-up medical care.

Occupational illness An infection or disease resulting from an occupational exposure; for example, an on-the-job- exposure to hepatitis B virus (an occupational exposure) can cause chronic hepatitis B disease (an occupational illness) in unvaccinated DHCP.

Occupational risk The chance of acquiring a disease through work-related circumstances.

OPIM See *Other potentially infectious materials.*

Other potentially infectious materials An Occupational Safety and Health Administration term that refers to body fluids or tissues that may contain bloodborne pathogens, or to body fluids that are visibly contaminated with blood. Abbreviated "OPIM."

Opportunistic infection An infection caused by a microorganism that does not ordinarily cause disease but can do so under certain host conditions (such as an immune disorder).

Oral surgical procedure The incision, excision, or reflection of tissue in the mouth that exposes areas of the oral cavity that normally are not exposed; examples include biopsy, periodontal surgery, apical surgery, implant surgery, and surgical extractions of teeth.

— P —

Parenteral Means of piercing the mucous membranes or the skin barrier through events such as a needlestick, human bite, cut, or abrasion.

Parenteral medication A medication delivered by piercing mucous membranes or the skin.

Pathogen Any microorganism that can cause disease in a host.

Patient-care item(s) Instruments and supplies used to provide dental examinations, prophylaxis, or treatment; examples include handpieces, cotton rolls, sutures, and air-water syringes.

Percutaneous injury An injury that penetrates the skin, such as a needlestick or a cut with a sharp object.

Persistent activity Prolonged or extended antimicrobial action that prevents or inhibits the growth or survival of microorganisms after a product has been used or applied; sometimes referred to as "residual activity."

Personal protective equipment Specialized clothing or devices worn by workers for protection against a hazard; in dentistry, includes gloves, mask, gown, and protective eyewear but not general work clothes (such as uniforms, pants, shirts, or blouses) that are not intended to protect against a hazard. Abbreviated "PPE."

Personal respiratory protection Disposable air-purifying respirator (for example, an N-95 respirator) worn to protect against exposure to airborne microorganisms; acts by filtering microscopic particles out of the air.

Plain soap A soap or detergent that contains no antimicrobial agents or very low concentrations of such agents that act only as a preservative.

Portal of entry A means of access to the body, for example, through the mucous membranes of the eyes, nose, or mouth; through a break in chapped skin; or through a cut or puncture wound.

Postexposure management The series of protocols recommended to minimize the chance of disease transmission after an occupational exposure; includes immediate reporting of the injury, preparing an exposure incident report, and referring the exposed individual to a qualified healthcare professional for evaluation, treatment, counseling and follow-up.

Postexposure prophylaxis The administration of medications or immunizations following an occupational exposure with the intent of preventing infection.

PPE See *Personal Protective Equipment.*

Preprocedural mouthrinse An antimicrobial mouthrinse used by a patient before treatment to reduce the number of microorganisms that can be released in aerosols or introduced into the patient's bloodstream during invasive dental procedures

Processing Patient-care items: The collection of actions that make contaminated instruments and other patient-care items safe for reuse on another patient; includes cleaning, inspection, packaging, heat sterilization, and storage and distribution.

Program evaluation Monitoring established infection control policies and procedures within a practice setting to ensure they are effective, properly implemented, and up to date.

Prosthesis A fixed or removable appliance that replaces missing teeth, for example, a bridge, denture, or partial.

Protective apparel Personal protective equipment: Garments that cover street clothes or uniforms to protect them from contamination during spatter-generating procedures; includes lab coats, clinic jackets, and gowns.

Protective eyewear Personal protective equipment: Impact-resistant safety glasses, goggles, or other eyewear with solid side shields that guard the eyes against splash, spatter, and debris.

— Q —

Qualified healthcare professional A physician or other healthcare professional who has the necessary and current training, expertise, and licensure to provide hepatitis B vaccination and postexposure evaluation and follow-up, including postexposure prophylaxis and counseling on the risks and possible consequences of occupational exposures.

— R —

Reflection The pushing or laying aside of tissue or an organ during surgery to gain access to the part to be operated on.

Regulated medical waste Waste generated through the delivery of medical or dental care that requires special handling and disposal because it can cause infection or physical harm (for example, blood- or saliva-soaked cotton rolls, extracted teeth, sharp items, surgically removed hard and soft tissues).

Resident flora Collection of microorganisms that are always present on or in the body and are not easily removed.

Retraction The drawing in of oral fluids or other debris from the mouth into dental waterlines or handpiece mechanisms, resulting in contamination that may be introduced to subsequent patients if equipment is not properly maintained or processed; also referred to as "suckback."

— S —

Safer medical devices See *Sharps safety devices.*

Self-contained water system A container attached to a dental unit that holds and supplies water or other solutions to handpieces and air-water syringes, isolating the unit from the public water system.

Semicritical Category of instruments or devices that contact but do not cut or penetrate mucous membranes.

Seroconversion The change of a serological test from negative to positive, indicating the development of antibodies in response to infection or immunization.

Sharps Objects that can cut or penetrate soft tissue; for example, needles, burs, explorers, endodontic files, broken anesthetic carpules.

Sharps safety device A device that incorporates features designed to reduce the risk of sharps injuries; examples include safety syringes, retractable scalpels, and needleless IV ports.

Shelf life Period of time a product or solution may be stored before use or activation without losing its effectiveness.

Single-use Intended to be used on one patient then discarded; not to be processed for reuse on another patient; disposable.

Source patient Exposure incident: The individual whose blood or other potentially infectious materials may be a source of occupational exposure.

Spatter Visible drops of liquid or body fluid that are expelled forcibly into the air and then quickly settle on nearby surfaces.

Specimen A portion or quantity of material for use in testing, examination, or study.

Standard precautions Practices and procedures that integrate and expand the elements of universal precautions into a standard of care designed to protect healthcare workers and patients from pathogens that can be spread by blood or any other body fluid, excretion, or secretion; applies to contact with blood; all body fluids, secretions, and excretions (except sweat), regardless of whether they contain blood; nonintact skin; and mucous membranes.

Sterilant A liquid chemical germicide that destroys all forms of microbiological life, including high numbers of resistant bacterial spores.

Sterile / sterility State of being free from all living microorganisms.

Sterile surgical gloves Sterile hand barriers than must be worn by DHCP during oral surgical procedures to protect the operating field from contamination and the operator's hands from exposure to the patient's blood and other fluid or tissue.

Sterile water Water that is free of microorganisms.

Sterile water delivery system A device or system that uses a reservoir and single-use disposable or sterilizable tubing to bypass the dental unit and deliver to the patient water or other solutions that are completely free of microorganisms

Sterilization The use of a physical (such as heat) or chemical procedure to destroy all microorganisms, including large numbers of resistant bacterial spores.

Sterilization monitoring Testing or observing heat-sterilization parameters using mechanical, chemical, and biological means. See *Biological monitoring, Chemical monitoring,* and *Mechanical monitoring.*

Substantivity The property of certain active ingredients that inhibits the growth of bacteria remaining on the skin.

Surfactant Agents that help cleaning by loosening, breaking down, and holding soil away from a surface so it can be more readily rinsed away.

Surgical hand antisepsis Preoperative antiseptic handwash or hand rub to eliminate transient and reduce resident microorganisms on the hands.

Surgical hand scrub A broad-spectrum, fast-acting, and persistent antiseptic-containing preparation that substantially reduces the number of microorganisms on intact skin.

Surgical procedure See *Oral surgical procedure.*

Surgical scrub The technique used to aseptically scrub hands before performing a surgical procedure.

Systemic Affecting the whole body.

— T —

Transient flora Microorganisms present on the outer layers of the skin for limited lengths of time; often acquired during direct contact with patients or contaminated environmental surfaces and relatively easy to remove by handwashing.

Transmission-based precautions Additional measures (that is, outside of standard precautions) necessary to prevent the spread of diseases that are transmitted through airborne, droplet, or contact transmission (for example, wearing an N-95 respirator to protect against tuberculosis transmission).

Treatment water See *Dental treatment water.*

Tuberculosis Disease caused by *Mycobacterium tuberculosis,* a bacterium that can infect various parts of the body but usually involves the lungs.

Active tuberculosis Contagious, usually symptomatic infection with *M. tuberculosis.*

Latent tuberculosis Condition in which *M. tuberculosis* is present in the body but the disease is not clinically active and the infected person is not contagious.

Tuberculocidal Able to destroy or irreversibly inactivate *Mycobacterium tuberculosis,* which is a test organism for disinfectant effectiveness; does not refer to prevention of tuberculosis transmission in the dental practice setting.

Type I hypersensitivity See *Anaphylaxis.*

Type IV hypersensitivity See *Allergic contact dermatitis.*

Ultrasonic cleaner Device that removes debris by a process called cavitation, in which waves of acoustic energy are generated in a solution to loosen and remove debris from objects.

Unit-dose Preparing and setting out supplies in the quantity needed before seating the patient; can minimize contact with and contamination of operatory surfaces during treatment.

Universal precautions A set of practices and procedures based on the concept that all blood and all body fluids that might be contaminated with blood should be treated as infectious; includes handwashing; use of engineering, work practice and administrative controls; and use of personal protective equipment.

Use life Germicides: Period of time a solution is effective after it has been opened, activated, or otherwise prepared for use.

Utility gloves Personal protective equipment: Heavy-duty, puncture-resistant, chemically resistant protection for the hands.

Vaccination Inoculation with a vaccine with the intent of producing immunity.

Vaccine A product administered through needle injections, by mouth, or by aerosol with the intent of producing immunity to protect the body against a disease.

Virus Submicroscopic organisms that infect cells, possibly causing disease.

Visibly soiled Showing evidence of blood, dirt, residual dental materials, or other debris.

Washer-disinfector An automatic device that uses a high-temperature cycle to clean and thermally disinfect instruments.

Waterless antiseptic agent See *Alcohol-based hand rub.*

Waterline The thin tubing that connects and carries treatment water from the water source (either the municipal water supply or a self-contained water system) to instruments used to treat patients.

Wicking Absorption of a liquid along a thread or through a material (for example, penetration of liquids through undetected holes in a glove).

Work practice controls Practices that reduce the likelihood of exposure by changing the manner in which a task is performed (for example, recapping needles with a one-handed scoop technique instead of using two hands).

Work restrictions / exclusions Limitations in professional duties as determined by policies set within the practice setting; may be imposed on DHCP whose health status poses a high risk of infection to patients, coworkers, or themselves.

Acknowledgments

OSAP thanks the following individuals for their contributions to *From Policy to Practice: OSAP's Guide to the CDC Guidelines*.

2019 Content Review Team

Kathy J. Eklund, RDH, MHP
The Forsyth Institute

Shellie Kolavic Gray, DMD, MPH
Consultant - Atlanta, GA

Ashley MacDermott, MPH, CHES
Organization for Safety, Asepsis and Prevention (OSAP)

Chris H. Miller, PhD
Indiana University School of Dentistry

Cover design by Neil Hinkle, Meeting Expectations. Additional photography appears courtesy of: Centers for Disease Control and Prevention (immunization, p. 13; tuberculin skin test series, p. 127); SmartPractice (occupational allergy, p. 41); Miele USA (instrument washer, p. 49); A-dec, Inc. (self-contained water system p. 76); DentaPure/MRLB (waterline filter, p. 76); Lares Research (sterile water delivery system, p. 76 and 111); Millipore (water sample test, p. 78, left); Pall Medical (water sample test, p. 78, right); USAF Dental Investigation Service (biofilm micrographs, p. 79 and 111); Eve Cuny, RDA, MS, University of the Pacific, (saliva ejector, p. 87 and 102; air-water syringe, p. 102; irrigating syringe, p. 111); Raghunath Puttaiah, BDS, MPH, Baylor College of Dentistry—TAMUS (x-ray film barrier series, p. 93); Crosstex (needle and syringe, p. 98); Septodont (anesthetic vial, p. 98); M. Joseph Olk, DDS (biopsy specimen series, p. 114); John A Molinari, PhD, University of Detroit Mercy (autoclave, p. 116).

Original Content Review Team

Helene Bednarsh, RDH, MPH
Eve Cuny, MS
Kathy J. Eklund, RDH, MHP
Therese M. Long, MBA, CAE
Donald W. Marianos, DDS, MPH
Shannon E. Mills, DDS
Charles J. Palenik, PhD, MS

Original Editorial and Production Team

Karen Ortolano
Karen Gomolka Editorial Services
Author / Editor / Art Director / Graphic Design / Production Manager

Scot Seguine
Illustrator

Mary Kay Gaydos
Clinical Photographer

M. Joseph Olk, DDS • Kathy Olk, RDH • Mindy Martin
M. Joseph Olk, DDS, PC
Clinical Models